Essentials in Ophthalmology

Series Editor
Arun D. Singh

For further volumes:
http://www.springer.com/series/5332

Colin Chan

Editor

Arun D. Singh

Series Editor

Dry Eye

A Practical Approach

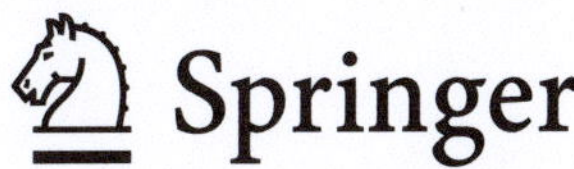 Springer

Editor
Colin Chan, MBBS (Hons) FRANZCO
Vision Eye Institute
School of Optometry and Vision Science
University of New South Wales
Sydney, NSW
Australia

Series Editor
Arun D. Singh
Department of Ophthalmic Oncology
Cole Eye Institute
Cleveland Clinic Foundation
Cleveland, OH
USA

ISSN 1612-3212
ISBN 978-3-662-52330-8   ISBN 978-3-662-44106-0   (eBook)
DOI 10.1007/978-3-662-44106-0
Springer Berlin Heidelberg New York Dordrecht London

Preface

On most working days, there will be a (usually female) distressed and sometimes crying patient sitting in front of me… telling about how dry eye is ruining her life. Why is this such a frequent scenario in my rooms? There are three reasons: (1) Dry eye affects all tasks of daily living, even sleep, and can impact severely the function and quality of life. (2) The incidence especially with the ageing population and increase in computer use is rising, and as dry eye persists and worsens without proper treatment, the prevalence is growing too. (3) Last, and the driving force behind this book, is the lack of sufficient understanding amongst the eyecare community on the appropriate treatment and management of dry eye patients.

This book aims to present current understanding of dry eye in an easy-to-read and practical manner. Key points are highlighted throughout each chapter, and each chapter is deliberately relatively short and to the point. A chapter of case reports enhances the practical teachings of the rest of the book. A look at the list of authors looks like a meeting of the United Nations. Each of the authors I know shares the same enthusiasm and passion for educating eyecare professionals in the treatment of dry eye.

I would like to thank these authors for their valuable contributions to this book. I would also like to thank Springer publications and their staff for bringing this book to publication. And, most importantly, I would like to thank my wife Amelia and my parents for their encouragement, love and support.

Sydney, NSW, Australia   Colin Chan, MBBS (Hons) FRANZCO

Contents

The Definition and Classification of Dry Eye Disease

Anthony J. Bron

1.1 Background

The tears occupy two compartments at the surface of the open eye. The first lies in the *fornices* and the spaces behind the lids, and the second is the *preocular tears*, comprising the *tear menisci* and the *tear film*. The precorneal part of the tear film is about 3 μm thick (King-Smith et al. 2000). Most of the aqueous component is derived from the lacrimal glands, a little from the conjunctiva, and gel mucin is added from the conjunctival goblet cells (Dartt 2002). Evaporation from the tear film is strongly retarded by its surface lipid layer, derived from the Meibomian glands. Water lost by evaporation is continuously replenished by newly formed tears, and fresh tears are regularly mixed and distributed by blinking and by eye movements. These actions protect the exposed ocular surface from desiccation. *Wettability* of the normal ocular surface is dependent on membrane-spanning mucins (MUC1, MUC4, and MUC16) present in the *glycocalyx* of the surface epithelial cells (Cope et al. 1986; Tiffany 1990a, b; Gipson et al. 2004), and two glycocalyx components, MUC16 and galactin-3,

are particularly important in excluding dye entry (fluorescein, lissamine green) into the healthy epithelium (Argüeso et al. 2006, 2009). Their absence is associated with punctate staining.

In sleep, when the eyes are closed, lacrimal secretion is at a minimum (Sack et al. 2000). In the waking state it is determined by sensory stimuli delivered to the exposed surface of the eye so that when the eyes open after sleep, the flow rate rises due to increased lacrimal secretion. Homeostasis of tear osmolarity is achieved by a reflex arc between the ocular surface and the secretory tissues, which regulates tear flow in response to adverse conditions. There is also a higher control centre responsible for emotional tears. The afferent limb of this reflex arc is provided by the trigeminal innervation of the ocular surface, particularly of the cornea, which is the most richly innervated tissue in the body (Rozsa and Beuerman 1982). The central processes of the trigeminal neurones synapse in the superior salivatory nucleus in the brainstem, where the efferent limb of the reflex arc arises, carried by the *nervus intermedius* of the VIIth cranial nerve. These parasympathetic fibres synapse with third-order neurones in the pterygopalatine ganglion, which supply the glandular tissues.

By means of this feedback loop, whose components comprise the lacrimal functional unit (LFU) (Stern et al. 1998, 2004), tear flow is adjusted in response to ambient conditions of air flow, temperature, and humidity. The LFU may be looked upon as a rapid response system, which

A.J. Bron, BSc, FRCOphth, FMedSci, FARVO
Nuffield Laboratory of Ophthalmology, Nuffield Department of Clinical Neurosciences,
University of Oxford and Oxford Eye Hospital, Oxford, UK

Vision and Eye Research Unit, Anglia Ruskin University, Cambridge, UK
e-mail: anthony.bron@eye.ox.ac.uk

C. Chan (ed.), *Dry Eye: A Practical Approach*, Essentials in Ophthalmology,
DOI 10.1007/978-3-662-44106-0_1, © Springer-Verlag Berlin Heidelberg 2015

compensates from moment to moment, for the effects of desiccating stress (e.g. low humidity and high wind speed) by an increase in tear flow and an increase in blink rate. Loss of this capacity makes an important contribution to the evolution of dry eye. Although goblet cells and Meibomian glands are innervated structures (Seifert and Spitznas 1999; Dartt 2002), there is no information as to how this reflex arc might regulate their secretions.

> The lacrimal functional unit (LFU) is a reflex-based system which controls the secretion of the aqueous and perhaps lipid and mucin components of tears in response to environmental stimuli.

1.2 The Definition of Dry Eye Disease

Medical definitions attempt to encapsulate the features of a disorder in order to distinguish it from other disorders. The task is difficult since diseases evolve over time, and a definition that fits one stage of the disease may not fit a later stage. Definitions are therefore an operational compromise, suited to some circumstances but not all. Classifications may be viewed in a similar way. They aim to group disorders according to their similarities. In this article, the definition of dry eye disease is based on the current understanding of its mechanism, and classification is based on how different aetiologies activate this mechanism.

At its simplest, dry eye disease is a chronic inflammatory condition of the ocular surface brought about by tear hyperosmolarity and usually accompanied by ocular surface symptoms. The ocular surface includes the surface of the cornea and of the bulbar and tarsal conjunctiva, extending to the lid margin. A recent international workshop (DEWS 2007a) provided the following definition:

> Dry eye is a multifactorial disease of the tears and ocular surface that results in symptoms of discomfort, visual disturbance and tear film instability, with potential damage to the ocular surface. It is accompanied by increased osmolarity of the tear film and inflammation of the ocular surface.

> - At its simplest, dry eye disease is a chronic inflammatory condition of the ocular surface brought about by tear hyperosmolarity and usually accompanied by ocular surface symptoms.
> - Like any chronic inflammatory condition, dry eye disease will continue to deteriorate if left untreated.
> - Lack of symptoms may not be a reason for withholding treatment.

1.3 Classification

The classification of dry eye disease is best understood by a consideration of its causes, that is, the manner by which tear hyperosmolarity is initiated and leads to ocular surface damage.

1.3.1 The Origins of Tear Hyperosmolarity

Tear hyperosmolarity may be brought about in two distinct ways, which are the basis of the two major classes of dry eye: (1) *aqueous-deficient dry eye* (ADDE) and (2) *evaporative dry eye* (EDE) (DEWS 2007a) (Fig. 1.1).

Aqueous-deficient dry eye is due to *lacrimal disease or dysfunction*, whereby tear hyperosmolarity is caused by evaporation from *a reduced volume of tears*. Reduced lacrimal secretion may come about from:

1. Organic disease of the lacrimal gland, as in Sjögren syndrome
2. Obstruction to its outflow, as in cicatricial pemphigoid
3. An interference with the homeostatic mechanism

In the latter case a reflex sensory blockade may be brought about by topical anaesthesia or trigeminal nerve section, and efferent blockade may result from damage to the pterygopalatine ganglion and third-order neurones (Slade et al. 1986). Additionally, lacrimal secretion may be inhibited pharmacologically by certain systemic drugs (Fraunfelder et al. 2012).

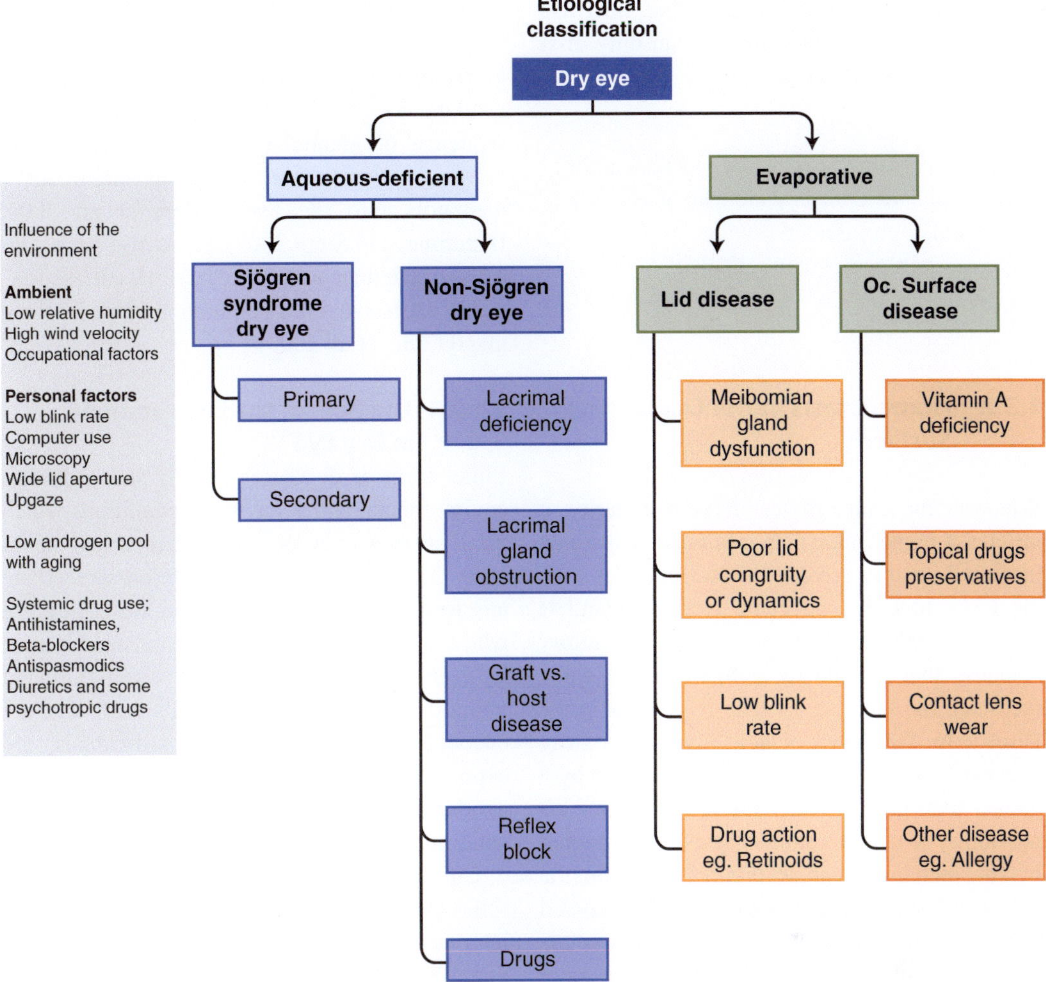

Fig. 1.1 Etiological classification of dry eye

There are two major classes of dry eye:
1. Aqueous-deficient dry eye
2. Evaporative dry eye

Both lead to tear hyperosmolarity.

Evaporative dry eye results from *increased evaporation* from the tear film in the presence of a normally functioning lacrimal gland. Since the tear film lipid layer is the major barrier to evaporation from the ocular surface, it is not surprising that Meibomian gland dysfunction (MGD), which causes a deficiency of the tear film lipid layer, is the chief cause of EDE. But evaporation can also be increased by a prolonged blink interval or a widened palpebral aperture, so that these too may cause EDE (Tsubota and Yamada 1992; Tsubota and Nakamori 1995).

MGD is the chief cause of evaporative dry eye.

It is important to recognise that, although the above distinction is clinically convenient, all forms of dry eye are in fact evaporative, since tear hyperosmolarity of consequence can only arise from evaporative water loss.

> Tear hyperosmolarity is key mechanism of both aqueous-deficient and evaporative dry eye and, with inflammation, is the primary driver of its pathogenic sequelae.

1.3.2 Homeostasis at the Ocular Surface

Whatever the cause of tear hyperosmolarity, it initiates a homeostatic response which causes an increased sensory drive to the lacrimal gland via the LFU. In EDE, since the lacrimal gland is healthy, this stimulates a lacrimal secretory response that is able to compensate, in some measure, for the rise in tear hyperosmolarity. Ultimately the level of tear hyperosmolarity reached in the steady state would be offset by a greater than normal tear volume and flow. This possibility of a high-volume dry eye is supported by the increased tear secretion (based on the Schirmer I test) in patients with MGD compared to normal (Shimazaki et al. 1995), although this evidence requires support by studies using more sophisticated tests of tear flow.

The same increase in sensory drive from the ocular surface would be expected in ADDE, but because of the basic lacrimal gland insufficiency, the level of osmolar compensation would be less, and in the steady state, this form of dry eye would be characterised by tear hyperosmolarity with a low tear volume and flow (Bron et al. 2009).

As an aside it may be noted that, experimentally, excessive reflex stimulation of the lacrimal gland may induce a *neurogenic inflammatory cytokine response* within the gland, leading to the sequence of glandular autoantigen expression, T-cell targeting, and the release of inflammatory mediators into the tears (Stern et al. 2004; Beuerman and Stern 2005). It has also been considered to induce a state of "lacrimal exhaustion" due to excessive reflex stimulation of the lacrimal gland (Tang et al. 2000).

1.3.2.1 The Role of the Environment in Dry Eye

Either form of disease is equally susceptible to environmental and behavioural conditions which can increase tear evaporation and raise tear osmolarity. These conditions can therefore exacerbate any form of dry eye or trigger its onset in those who are predisposed. These circumstances arise in everyday life in situations where ambient humidity is low or wind speeds high and are encountered regularly when individuals are exposed to air conditioning and/or high altitude, as during air travel, or in adverse climatic conditions.

Similarly, evaporation is increased by personal factors, which may be looked upon as the internal environment. Thus, tear hyperosmolarity may be induced by an extended blink interval or a widened palpebral aperture, which occur during VDT use, reading, microscopy and the performance of difficult visual tasks which reduce the blink rate, or extended periods with the eyes held up in gaze, as when searching for goods on high shelves in the supermarket or when playing games like snooker. Additionally, systemic drugs which reduce lacrimal secretion are a potential cause of tear hyperosmolarity and may be a risk

> Both ADDE and EDE lead to an increased reflex drive to the lacrimal gland. In EDE, the lacrimal gland responds sufficiently to compensate at least initially; in ADDE, it cannot.

> Evaporation may be increased by environmental factors such as:
> - Wind/air conditioning
> - Prolonged visual attention, e.g. computer use, reading

factor for dry eye (DEWS 2007b-Epidemiology). The relationship between activities of daily living and the symptoms of dry eye disease has been explored by Iyer et al. (2012).

Some of these factors play an important part in the symptoms of dry eye that occur in the workplace and affect, for instance, office workers and airline staff. Vulnerability to such exposure may influence suitability for work or the outcome of surgery, such as LASIK. Knowledge of such influences may allow preventative measures to be devised and instituted.

1.3.2.2 Hyperosmolarity: The Proximate Cause Dry Eye

Tear hyperosmolarity is regarded as the central mechanism of any form of dry eye disease, occurring either directly, as a response to reduced tear flow or increased tear evaporation, or indirectly, as a result of tear film instability. Once tear hyperosmolarity is established at the surface of the eye, it gives rise to a vicious circle of events that results, initially, in symptoms and compensatory responses but also in inflammatory responses, chronic ocular surface damage and ultimately in self-perpetuated disease (Baudouin 2007; DEWS 2007a).

Tear hyperosmolarity stimulates a cascade of inflammatory events in the epithelial cells of the ocular surface, involving MAP kinases and NF-kB signalling pathways (Li et al. 2004) and the generation of inflammatory cytokines (IL-1α, IL-1β, TNF-α) and MMPs (e.g. MMP9) (De Paiva et al. 2006). These arise from or activate inflammatory cells at the ocular surface (Baudouin 2001) and lead to reduced expression of glycocalyx mucins, apoptotic death of surface epithelial cells and loss of goblet cells (Yeh et al. 2003). Epithelial cell damage or death is the basis for ocular surface staining in dry eye and is contributed to by loss of glycocalyx mucins, which removes a barrier for dye entry and which also compromises ocular surface wetting (Bron et al. 2015). Goblet cell loss is a feature of every form of dry eye (Kunert et al. 2002; Brignole et al. 2000), demonstrable by conjunctival biopsy and impression cytology and reflected by reduced levels of the gel mucin MUC5AC (Zhao et al. 2001; Argüeso et al. 2002).

> Once tear hyperosmolarity is established at the surface of the eye, it gives rise to a *vicious circle of events* that results, initially, in symptoms and compensatory responses but also to in inflammatory responses, chronic ocular surface damage and ultimately to in *self-perpetuated disease*

These events contribute to the clinical picture of dry eye in a number of ways, by stimulating sensory nerve endings in the cornea and to a lesser extent the conjunctiva. Symptoms of discomfort can be caused by tear hyperosmolarity, algaesic inflammatory mediators and by increased shear stress imparted during blinking and eye movements with loss of the lubricative goblet cell mucin. Surface damage, and particularly the loss of the epithelial glycocalyx, leads to defective wettability, tear film instability and to a progressive shortening of the tear film break-up time until a point is reached when break-up occurs within the blink interval. This is a potential turning point in the evolution of any form of dry eye, since tear break-up itself initiates a wave of hyperosmolarity which spreads across the corneal surface as the zone of break-up expands and whose peak is located at the origin of the break-up (Peng et al. 2014). The shorter the break-up time, the greater the level of local hyperosmolarity achieved and the longer the period of exposure of the eye to this hyperosmolarity.

Tear break-up in the blink interval is the event which completes the *vicious circle* in the mechanism of dry eye and perpetuates the disease (Baudouin 2007). Break-up augments hyperosmolar surface damage and, in turn, increased damage causes greater tear film instability; this amplifies the hyperosmolarity and so on. In this way it is thought that dry eye can become a semi-autonomous condition, in which the initiating cause could play a secondary role.

> Tear break-up within the blink interval is the tipping point of dry eye. This augments the hyperosmolar surface damage, which then leads to even greater tear instability.

More importantly, stimulation of trigeminal nerve terminals, in addition to causing pain, is responsible for compensatory events in dry eye, acting through the LFU, such as increased lacrimal secretion and blink rate, which tend to offset the development of tear hyperosmolarity (Tsubota 1998). These influence the clinical features of dry eye and are dealt with in a later section dealing with hybrid forms of dry eye.

1.4 An Etiological Classification of Dry Eye (Fig. 1.1)

1.4.1 Aqueous-Deficient Dry Eye

1.4.1.1 Sjögren Syndrome Dry Eye (SSDE)

Sjögren syndrome is an *exocrinopathy* in which the lacrimal and salivary glands are targeted by a widespread autoimmune process. Other organ systems are also affected. The lacrimal and salivary glands are infiltrated by activated T-cells, which cause acinar and ductular cell death and hyposecretion of tears or saliva. Inflammatory activation within the glands leads to the expression of autoantigens at the surface of epithelial cells (e.g. fodrin, Ro and La) (Nakamura et al. 2006) and the retention of tissue-specific CD4[+] and CD8[+] T-cells (Hayashi et al. 2003). Salivary gland infiltration ranges from scattered T-cell invasion in mild disease, to diffuse inflammation in severe disease, with B-cells predominating and with progressive loss of glandular tissue. Historically, Th1 cells and their products such as INF Υ were considered to be the chief instruments of tissue damage, but there is now evidence for a major role for Th-17 cells (T follicular (Tf), Th22 and Treg cells – the IL-17 axis) and their products, especially IL-17, in the salivary and lacrimal glands (Alunno et al. 2014; Zhang et al. 2012). Hyposecretion is amplified by a potentially reversible neurosecretory block due to the effects of locally released inflammatory cytokines or to the presence of circulating antibodies (e.g. anti-M3) (Zoukhri 2006; Dawson et al. 2006). Sjögren syndrome is termed secondary when it is part of a defined autoimmune or connective tissue disorder such as rheumatoid arthritis, systemic lupus erythematosis, scleroderma, primary biliary sclerosis and dermatomyositis. Rheumatoid Sjögren syndrome is the commonest form. Primary Sjögren syndrome is an autoimmune disorder in its own right.

Sjögren syndrome is not uncommonly accompanied by Meibomian gland dysfunction (MGD) which is a potential cause of evaporative dry eye so that the dry eye in these patients may include an interaction between ADDE and EDE (Shimazaki et al. 1998).

1.4.1.2 Non-Sjögren Syndrome Dry Eye (NSDE)

Primary Lacrimal Deficiencies

Non-Sjögren syndrome dry eye (NSDE) is any form of ADDE due to lacrimal disease or dysfunction where systemic autoimmune features, characteristic of SSDE, have been excluded. However, unless otherwise stated, the term NSDE will be used here to refer to age-related lacrimal deficiency (see below).

Congenital Alacrima

Congenital alacrima or lacrimal agenesis may occur as an inherited disorder (Hegab and al-Mutawa 1996) sometimes with agenesis of the salivary glands (Kim et al. 2005) and is a rare cause of dry eye in youth or infancy. It may also occur as part of an inherited syndrome (see below).

Lacrimal Gland Ablation

Dry eye may be caused by ablation of the lacrimal gland at any age or by severance of the ducts, which enter into the superolateral fornix, during lid surgery. Dry eye is not an inevitable outcome, since the accessory glands and conjunctival secretions may compensate in some cases (Scherz and Dohlman 1975).

Age-Related Lacrimal Gland Deficiency

Age-related lacrimal gland deficiency is the commonest form of NSDE and is encountered chiefly in older subjects. In the past it was referred to as keratoconjunctivitis sicca (KCS) (Lemp 1995; DEWS 2007a). With ageing, in the normal population, there is an increasing infiltration of lacrimal glands with CD4[+] and CD8[+] T-cells, leading to a gradual destruction of lacrimal acinar and ductal cells and a reduction in lacrimal secretion. Histopathologically, a low-grade dacryoadenitis leads to periductal fibrosis, interacinar fibrosis, paraductal blood vessel loss and acinar cell atrophy (Obata 2006). The clinical features resemble those of SSDE, but, in general, its age of onset is later, its rate of progression slower and its severity generally less marked than in SSDE.

Secondary Lacrimal Gland Deficiencies

Alacrima

Alacrima may occur as part of an inherited syndrome.

(i) *Triple A or Allgrove syndrome*. Triple A or Allgrove syndrome is a progressive, recessively inherited disorder, in which congenital alacrima is associated with achalasia of the cardia, Addison's disease, a central neurodegeneration and autonomic dysfunction. It is caused by mutations in the AAAS gene, encoding the protein ALADIN (Brooks et al. 2005; Sarathi and Shah 2010).

(ii) *Familial Dysautonomia (Riley–Day Syndrome)*. *Familial dysautonomia (Riley-Day syndrome)* is an autosomal recessive disorder due to mutations in a gene encoding an IkB kinase-associated protein (Gold-von Simson and Axelrod 2006).

Dry eye and corneal damage are major features of the disorder, with a marked lack of emotional and reflex tearing and a loss of sensory innervation of the ocular surface. There is a congenital, generalised insensitivity to pain. Lacrimal dysfunction is caused by a loss of autonomic innervation to the lacrimal gland.

Alacrima can also be associated with blepharophimosis (Athappilly and Braverman 2009), lacrimal-auriculo-dental-digital syndrome (LADD) and Pierre Robin sequence.

Lacrimal Gland Infiltration

In certain systemic diseases, tear secretion may be reduced by other forms of inflammatory infiltration of the lacrimal gland.

(i) *Sarcoidosis*. Dry eye is caused by infiltration of the lacrimal gland with sarcoid granulomata (James et al. 1964).

(ii) *Lymphoma*. Here, dry eye is due to an infiltration by lymphomatous cells (Heath 1949).

(iii) *AIDS*. AIDS-related dry eye is caused by T-cell infiltration of the lacrimal gland, predominantly by CD8[+] suppressor cells, unlike the situation in SSDE, where CD4[+] helper cells are involved (Itescu et al. 1990).

Graft Versus Host Disease (GVHD)

Dry eye is a common complication of GVHD disease, occurring typically around 6 months after haematopoietic stem cell transplantation (Ogawa and Kuwana 2003). Immune attack is directed to the lacrimal glands and to the whole of the ocular surface. As a result, a complex, combined form of dry eye occurs, with features of both ADDE and EDE and additionally, ocular surface inflammation due to the primary disease itself. Lacrimal gland fibrosis is due to the co-localization of periductal T-lymphocytes (CD4[+] and CD8[+]) with antigen-presenting fibroblasts in the glands (Ogawa et al. 2003). Evaporative dry eye results from cicatricial MGD and is associated with extensive Meibomian gland atrophy and drop-out (Ban et al. 2011).

Lacrimal Gland Duct Obstruction

Obstruction of the ducts of the main, palpebral and accessory lacrimal glands by scar tissue may occur with any form of cicatrising conjunctivitis, causing a secondary ADDE. The scarring process may, in addition, cause a cicatricial form of MGD, so that an evaporative component is added to the dry eye and this may be exacerbated by lid deformity with its consequent effects on aqueous dynamics.

Conditions giving rise to lacrimal duct obstruction include trachoma, cicatricial pemphigoid and mucous membrane pemphigoid, erythema multiforme and chemical and thermal burns.

Reflex Block

This refers to a reduction in lacrimal secretion due to interference with the reflex arc of the LFU. Lacrimal tear secretion in the waking state is maintained by a trigeminal sensory drive arising chiefly from the cornea, probably arising, in particular, from the cold modality sensory fibres. When the eyes are closed, as during sleep, lacrimal secretion is at its lowest, since the sensory input falls to a minimum. When the eyes are open, there is an increased reflex sensory drive from the exposed ocular surface.

(i) Afferent Blockade. A reduction in sensory drive from the ocular surface is thought to favour the occurrence of dry eye in two ways: first, by decreasing reflex-induced lacrimal secretion and, second, by reducing the blink rate and, hence, increasing evaporative loss in the blink interval. Bilateral, topical proparacaine decreases the blink rate by about 30 % and tear secretion by 60–75 % (Jordan and Baum 1980).

In addition, it has recently been found that tear osmolarity is influenced by the internal environment and reflects the level of body hydration. Thus, plasma osmolarity is increased in patients with dry eye, and increased tear osmolality and, conversely, tear osmolarity is increased in patients with decreased body hydration, a condition that is not uncommon in the aged and may be life threatening (Fortes et al. 2011; Walsh et al. 2012). There is therefore an interest in using tear osmolarity to detect body dehydration, since the measurement of tear osmolality is a quick and reliable test.

(ii) *Efferent blockade.* Parasympathetic denervation of the human lacrimal gland may result from a peripheral, VIIth cranial nerve palsy involving the *N. intermedius* (Tamura et al. 2008), which may, for instance, follow surgery for acoustic neuroma. Since the main palpebral and accessory glands are similarly innervated, there is no opportunity for secretory compensation. Furthermore, since the VIIth nerve palsy causes lagophthalmos, there will be an additional exposure element to the keratopathy due to incomplete or absent lid closure.

1.4.2 Evaporative Dry Eye

Evaporative dry eye results from an excessive rate of evaporation from the ocular surface in the presence of normal lacrimal function. Its causes may be *lid-related* or *ocular surface-related* (Fig. 1.1), also referred to as intrinsic and extrinsic EDE, respectively.

1.4.2.1 Lid-Related Evaporative Dry Eye
Meibomian Gland Dysfunction
The Meibomian glands are embedded in the tarsal plates, and their orifices lie just anterior to the mucocutaneous junction. Meibomian oil is delivered onto the skin of the free margin of the lid from whence it is spread onto the surface of the tear film in the up-phase of each blink.

Meibomian gland dysfunction (MGD) is the most common cause of evaporative dry eye (Foulks and Bron 2003; Bron and Tiffany 2004; Bron et al. 2004). It was recently defined at the International Workshop on MGD as follows, and further details may be found in that report (Nichols et al. 2011; Nelson et al. 2011):

> Meibomian gland dysfunction (MGD) is a chronic, diffuse abnormality of the meibomian glands, commonly characterised by terminal duct obstruction and/or qualitative/quantitative changes in the glandular secretion. This may result in alteration of the tear film, symptoms of eye irritation, clinically apparent inflammation, and ocular surface disease.

MGD may be primary or secondary to other local ocular or systemic diseases. Cicatricial and non-cicatricial forms exist (Foulks and Bron 2003) (Fig. 1.2). In primary MGD, there is no associated local or systemic disease.

Non-Cicatricial MGD
In *non-cicatricial MGD*, probably the commonest form of MGD, the terminal ducts are obstructed by a process of hyperkeratinisation and possibly by increased lipid viscosity. The gland orifices remain located in the skin of the lid margin, anterior to the mucocutaneous junction (Jester et al. 1989a, b; Knop et al. 2011). This has therapeutic implications, since, if gland function can be restored, the orifices are in the proper position for oil delivery. Obstruction is accompanied by a thickening and clouding of expressed Meibomian secretions (meibum), which blocks the ducts and may cause plugging of the orifices. Obstruction leads to secondary gland atrophy, which appears as gland "drop out" on meibography. Non-cicatricial MGD most commonly occurs as a primary disorder, seen with increasing frequency after the age of 50 years. It also has multiple secondary associations, including dermatoses such as rosacea, seborrhoeic dermatitis and atopic dermatitis (McCulley and Sciallis 1977; McCulley et al. 1982). Additionally, it should be noted that the retinoid, isotretinoin, used in the treatment of acne vulgaris causes reversible Meibomian gland atrophy, with features

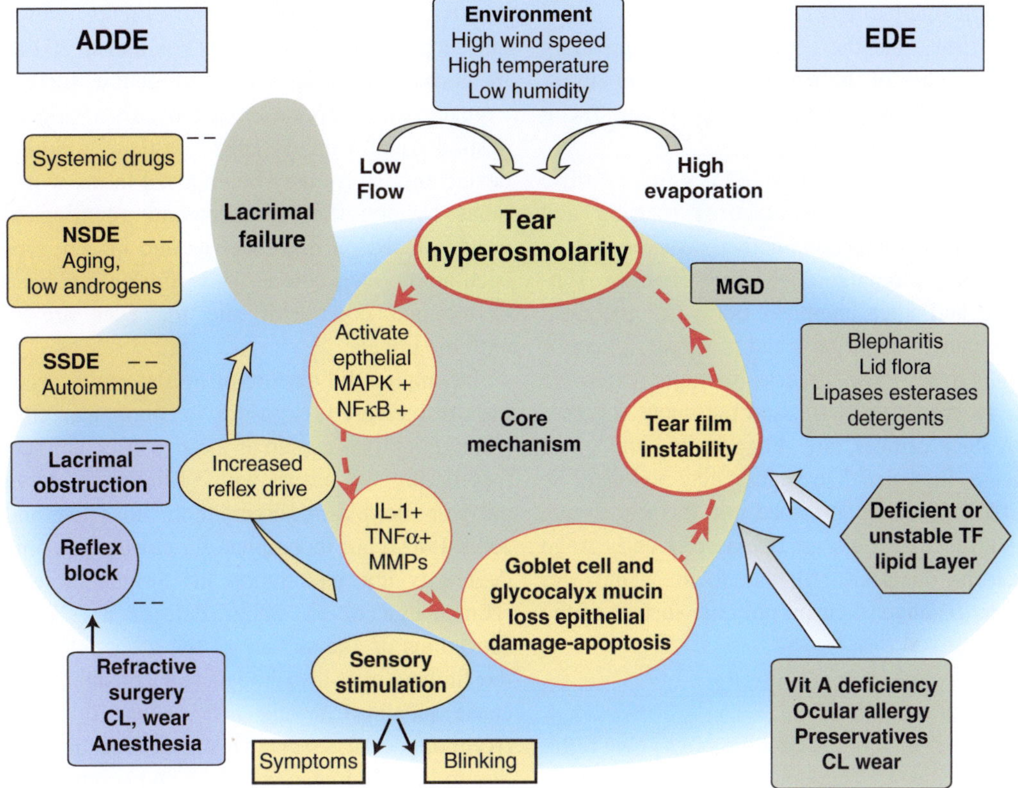

Fig. 1.2 Mechanisms of dry eye

of MGD (Fraunfelder et al. 1985; Mathers et al. 1991a). Also, occurring in rare epidemics, systemic exposure to polychlorinated biphenyls, through ingestion of contaminated cooking oils, has caused a chronic disorder with gross and extensive acneiform skin changes, Meibomian seborrhoea with thick excreta and glandular cyst formation (Ohnishi et al. 1975; Fu 1984).

- Meibomian gland atrophy is the end result of chronic MGD.
- Therefore:
- The current MGD guidelines recommend proactive treatment even if minimal symptoms are present to prevent Meibomian gland damage.
- Some patients with end-stage MGD and atrophic Meibomian glands may be unresponsive to treatment.

Cicatricial MGD

In primary, cicatricial MGD, duct obstruction is due to an elongation, stretching and narrowing of the terminal ducts and due to a very local conjunctival scarring process in the region of the terminal duct and orifice. As a result, each affected orifice and associated duct is dragged from its position anterior to the mucocutaneous junction into the neighbouring marginal conjunctival mucosa. The key diagnostic feature is the presence of tell-tale *elevated ridges* in the occlusal mucosa of the free margin of the lid, which represent the dragged terminal ducts exposed under a thinned mucosal epithelium. Cicatricial MGD may affect scattered glands, in the same lid, in conjunction with non-cicatricial MGD (see below).

In non-cicatricial MGD, diagnosis is based on the morphologic features of the gland acini and duct orifices; the presence of orifice plugging, thickening and clouding or absence of expressed excreta. Methods exist to grade the degree of MGD (Bron et al. 1991; Mathers et al. 1991b) and measure the degree of gland dropout (meibography) (Mathers et al. 1991b; Arita et al. 2008, 2010), the amount of oil in the lid margin reservoir (meibometry) (Chew et al. 1993; Yokoi et al. 1999) and the appearance and spreading characteristics of the tear film lipid layer (interferometry) (Yokoi et al. 1996; Goto and Tseng 2003).

Secondary, cicatricial MGD is a more diffuse process caused by conjunctival scarring and occurs in cicatricial conjunctival diseases such as trachoma, pemphigoid, Stevens-Johnson syndrome and after chemical burns. It may also accompany rosacea and vernal keratoconjunctivitis. The process is more extensive than in primary disease, and the ducts, together with their orifices, are dragged into the tarsal mucosa. In severe disease they may no longer be visible as they are absorbed into the scar tissue. In both forms of disease, even at an early stage when the ducts are still patent, the glands are unable to deliver their oil onto the surface of the tear film.

The Symptoms of MGD

MGD is a symptomatic condition in its own right, which can be associated with a normal tear evaporation rate (Shimazaki et al. 1995). However, with progression of the disease, the degree and extent of obstruction results in a tear film lipid layer deficiency and loss of its barrier function to evaporation (Craig and Tomlinson 1997). Contributing factors are thinning and irregularity of the Tear Film Lipid Layer (TFLL), a reduced spread time with each blink and probably, lipid compositional changes (Foulks et al. 2010). This leads to an increase in tear evaporation rate, which ultimately may cause evaporative dry eye (Mathers 1993; Mathers et al. 1996; Shimazaki et al. 1995, 1998; Goto et al. 2003; Tomlinson and Khanal 2005).

Disorders of Lid Aperture and Lid/Globe Congruity or Dynamics

An increase in palpebral fissure width or globe prominence exposes the tear film to greater evaporation (Gilbard and Farris 1983) and the risk of ocular desiccation and tear hyperosmolarity. In Graves' disease the effect of proptosis on exposure is compounded by lid retraction and lid lag, incomplete blinking or lid closure and by restriction of eye movements, which plays a part in tear spreading (Yokoi et al. 2014). In normal subjects, increased ocular surface exposure and evaporation also occurs in upgaze (Tsubota and Yamada 1992), so that, as noted, desiccating stress may be imposed in the workplace by activities that demand attention to goods placed on high shelves and in activities such as snooker, where, while aiming, the head is inclined downward and the eyes are in extreme upgaze.

Incomplete lid closure or lid deformity, leading to increased exposure or poor tear film resurfacing, is accepted as a cause of ocular surface drying and occurs with VIIth cranial nerve palsy or after plastic surgery to the lids (Rees and Jelks 1981), but incomplete lid closure of some degree is not uncommon in normal subjects (Himebaugh et al. 2009; Pult et al. 2013). Elevations on the surface of the globe, close to the limbus, may also impair tear spreading and cause localised drying and dellen formation (Kymionis et al. 2011). This may occur in relation to local tumours, chemosis and conjunctival haemorrhage, with filtering blebs, after pterygium, strabismus and cataract surgery and in Graves' disease.

Low Blink Rate

Drying of the ocular surface may be caused by a reduced blink rate, which lengthens the blink interval and extends the period for evaporation of tears before the next blink (Abelson and Holly 1977; Collins et al. 2006). Reduced blink rate may occur during tasks involving increased concentration, e.g. working at video terminals (Nakamori et al. 1997), with video games, and at microscopes, and also occurs when the eyes are in downgaze, as in reading. It also accompanies the extrapyramidal disorder Parkinson's disease (PD), where it may be the basis for dry eye and in progressive ophthalmoplegia, where, in addition, the spreading of tears is impaired by a reduction in eye movements. Other contributing factors in PD may be reduced Meibomian oil delivery, decreased reflex tearing due to autonomic dysfunction (Magalhaes et al. 1995), and the effects of androgen deficiency on the lacrimal and Meibomian glands (Okun et al. 2002).

1.4.2.2 Ocular Surface Related Disorders: Extrinsic Causes

Disease of the exposed ocular surface may lead to imperfect surface wetting, early tear film break-up, tear hyperosmolarity, and dry eye. Causes include vitamin A deficiency and the effects of chronically applied topical anaesthetics and preservatives. Contact lenses may be responsible for increased water loss from the eye.

Vitamin A Deficiency

In vitamin A deficiency, (xerophthalmia), dry eye is caused by a reduction in conjunctival goblet cell numbers and a reduced expression of glycocalyx mucins (Tei et al. 2000), leading to an unstable tear film and a reduced tear break-up time. In addition, damage to the lacrimal gland may result in a true aqueous-deficient dry eye (Sommer and Emran 1982).

Topical Drugs and Preservatives

Topical drugs and preservatives can induce an inflammatory response at the ocular surface, leading to dry eye (Rolando et al. 1991). Glaucoma patients, receiving preserved drops on a long-term basis, particularly benzalkonium chloride, are especially at risk (Jaenen et al. 2007). In an unmasked study of 4,107 glaucoma patients, ocular surface changes were twice as common in those receiving preserved drops than in those receiving unpreserved drops, and the frequency of signs and symptoms was dose related but reversible on switching to unpreserved preparations (Pisella et al. 2002). Short-term exposure to preservative can reduce tear film stability and increase epithelial permeability (Ishibashi et al. 2003). In the longer term, the chain of events appears to be that inflammatory events, e.g. signified by increased HLA-DR and ICAM-1 expression, lead to cell damage and apoptotic death and epitheliopathy, including goblet cell loss, reduced MUC5AC expression and poor ocular surface wettability (Baudouin et al. 1999, 2010). Fraunfelder has drawn attention to the multiple ways in which systemic or topical polypharmacy may interact and give rise to dry eye disease (Fraunfelder et al. 2012).

Topical Anaesthesia

Topical anaesthesia causes drying in two ways. It reduces lacrimal secretion by reducing sensory drive to the lacrimal gland (Jordan and Baum 1980) and also reduces the blink rate. Chronic use of topical anaesthetics can cause a neurotrophic keratitis and lead to corneal perforation (Pharmakakis et al. 2002; Chen et al. 2004).

Contact Lens Wear

Chronic contact lens (CL) wear may induce epithelial changes (Knop and Brewitt 1992) and the expression of inflammatory surface markers (HLA-DR and ICAM-1) (Pisella et al. 2001). The effect on goblet cell density (Connor et al. 1994, 1997; Lievens et al. 2003) and mucin expression (Pisella et al. 2001; Hori et al. 2006) has varied in different studies. Nonetheless, about 50 % of CL wearers report dry eye symptoms (Doughty et al. 1997; Begley et al. 2000, 2001), which are about 12 times more likely than in emmetropes and five times more likely than in spectacle wearers (Nichols et al. 2005). Women report dry eye symptoms more frequently than men (Nichols and Sinnott 2006). Dry eye symptoms in contact lens wearers are associated with a higher tear osmolarity, but not in the range normally associated with dry eye tear hyperosmolarity (Nichols and Sinnott 2006). Although there are conflicting reports (Cedarstaff and Tomlinson 1983; Schlanger 1993; Fonn et al. 1999), in general it is accepted that high water content lenses are associated with a thinner tear film lipid layer, a faster tear film thinning time, a higher evaporative water loss and a greater likelihood of dry eye symptoms. Poor lens wettability may also play a part in the increased evaporation. Efron et al. found that patients wearing low-water CLs, which maintained their hydration, were free from symptoms (Efron and Brennan 1988). Conversely, various studies suggest that features compatible with a dry eye state may predispose an individual to CL intolerance (Glasson et al. 2003).

Allergic Conjunctivitis

Allergic conjunctivitis takes several forms, which include seasonal allergic conjunctivitis (SAC), vernal keratoconjunctivitis (VKC) and atopic keratoconjunctivitis (AKC). Ocular allergy was noted to be a risk factor for dry eye in the Beaver Dam Study, even after adjustment for concomitant use of systemic medications, such as antihistamines (Moss et al. 2004, 2008). In SAC, exposure to antigen in sensitised subjects leads to degranulation of IgE-primed mast cells, with the release of inflammatory cytokines. A Th2 response is activated at the ocular surface, initially in the conjunctival and, later, in the corneal epithelium. Experimentally, there is stimulation of goblet cell secretion and loss of surface membrane mucins (Kunert et al. 2001). Surface epithelial cell death occurs, leading to punctate keratoconjunctivitis. Surface damage and the release of inflammatory mediators lead to allergic symptoms.

In VKC and AKC there are additional inflammatory and submucosal changes. Surface irregularities on the cornea and conjunctiva can lead to tear film instability and a local drying component to the allergic eye disease. This may be amplified by MGD (Ibrahim et al. 2012). Lid swelling and lid margin irregularity can interfere with lid apposition and tear film spreading, thus exacerbating the dry eye.

1.5 Symptoms, Hybrid States and Complex Forms of Dry Eye

1.5.1 Sources of Symptoms

Established dry eye is a symptomatic disorder that frequently gives rise to chronic disability. But patients may be encountered in whom ocular surface staining, early tear break-up and even tear hyperosmolarity may be found by chance in the absence of symptoms. There is insufficient knowledge of the natural history of dry eye to know what the long-term clinical outcome might be in such individuals. Nonetheless, there is evidence that patients with "incomplete dry eye"

may suffer worse outcomes following refractive surgery procedures, including a greater risk of refractive regression (Goto et al. 2004). It is therefore important to identify such patients in order make surgical decisions and to give prognostic advice.

It is important to identify dry eye even if the patient is asymptomatic as dry eye may affect:
- Refractive surgery outcomes
- Contact lens tolerance

Similarly, MGD is thought of as a symptomatic disease but may exist in an asymptomatic form without clinically visible lid margin or ocular surface signs. Korb has termed this condition, which is detectable only on the basis of abnormal expressability or quality of meibum on gland expression, as "nonobvious" MGD (Blackie et al. 2010). Again it is not known whether, in the absence of treatment, this form of the disease will give rise to chronic, symptomatic MGD in the longer term or even to MGD-related evaporative dry eye. Nonetheless, it is likely that it represents a risk factor for contact lens intolerance in those considering contact lens wear.

Symptoms of dry eye are due to pathological events at the ocular surface, and yet it is often observed that there is a poor correlation between the symptoms of dry eye and objectively recorded signs (Begley et al 2003; Nichols et al. 2004; Sullivan et al. 2014). This is particularly problematic in relation to clinical trials, when the ability to suppress some clinical signs of the disease is not accompanied by a reduction in symptoms. There are many possible reasons for this mismatch, the most likely of which is that there are multiple events that contribute to discomfort and that their relative contribution to symptoms changes during the evolution of the disease. Thus, since tear hyperosmolarity is the core element of classical dry eye and hyperosmolar solutions instilled topically can induce pain (Liu et al. 2009), tear hyperosmolarity would be expected to provide an early basis for pain in this condition. If this were the only source of pain in dry eye, however, then simple closure of the eye to prevent evaporation would relieve the discomfort of the eye within a short space of time, which is not the case.

Stimulation of the ocular surface by hyperosmolarity leads to the release of inflammatory mediators into the tears, some of which have algaesic properties and may stimulate sensory nerve endings. Examples include prostaglandins, cytokines and neurokinins. It has also been mentioned that, with increasing severity of dry eye, there is a progressive fall in goblet cell density and therefore the expectation that ocular surface lubrication will suffer. This gives rise to the expectation of symptoms resulting from frictional drag between the apposed surfaces of the eye, of the lids and the globes. To this may be added symptoms that may originate in conditions associated with dry eye, either from an initiating disease, such as MGD, which is itself symptomatic, or from a disorder apparently secondary to the dry eye, such as conjunctivochalasis (Di Pascuale et al. 2004; Yokoi et al. 2005) or lid wiper epitheliopathy (Korb et al. 2005, 2010).

> The mismatch between symptoms and signs in dry eye may be because multiple factors contribute to "dry eye pain" such as:
> - Tear hyperosmolarity
> - Release of algaesic inflammatory mediators
> - Frictional drag between lids and the conjunctiva caused by loss of goblet cells
> - Change in corneal sensation

1.5.2 The Role of Corneal Sensitivity

The natural history of corneal sensitivity is incompletely known in dry eye but is relevant to the occurrence of both symptoms and compensatory responses. Increased corneal sensory excitability has been recorded in dry eye patients (De Paiva and Pflugfelder 2004) or subjects with dry eye symptoms (Situ et al. 2008) which would be expected to enhance both pain and the compensatory lacrimal response to noxious stimuli. Most reports, however (Xu et al. 1996; Bourcier et al. 2005), suggest that corneal sensitivity is impaired in chronic dry eye disease. Certainly, morphological changes have been recorded in dry eye disease by confocal microscopy, including a reduction in sub-basal nerve plexus bundles (Benitez-Del-Castillo et al. 2007). It is tempting to advance the notion that as the severity of dry eye progresses, it goes through a stage: first of sensory hyper-excitability and then of sensory depression. At this stage of dry eye, the reflex sensory drive to lacrimal secretion would become reduced, which would reverse any compensatory drive to lacrimal secretion that is postulated for the earlier phase of the disease. This could result in a reduction of symptoms but would have consequences for the clinical phenotype of the disease (Bron et al. 2009).

1.5.3 Hybrid Forms of Dry Eye

Since MGD is a common disorder, which may become extensive, it is not uncommon for ADDE and EDE to occur together, in which case the severity of the resulting dry eye is increased. An obvious example is in SSDE (Shimazaki et al. 1995). Also, mixed forms of dry eye were common in a recent multicentre study of dry eye (Lemp et al. 2012). In these examples the hybrid dry eye disease results from the co-existence of two, organic forms of disease occurring in combination. However, hybrid forms may come about in other ways.

It has been proposed that, in the early stages of dry eye, ocular surface changes result in an increased sensory drive to the lacrimal gland, resulting in a differential compensatory response in different forms of ADDE and EDE. For instance it is predicted that in MGD-related EDE, there is initially an unrestricted lacrimal response to this sensory input from the healthy lacrimal gland. The rising level of tear osmolarity would result in an increased lacrimal flow and tear volume, which would offset the steady-state level of hyperosmolarity (Tung et al. 2014). With advancing disease, sensory loss at the ocular surface, by reducing sensory drive, would reduce this compensation, and tear hyperosmolarity would rise in direct proportion to the fall in lacrimal flow. This would give rise to a hybrid condition of organic

EDE due to MGD combined with a functional ADDE due to a loss of LFU compensation.

By comparison, in the case of organic ADDE, there is a progressive fall in lacrimal secretion due to advancing lacrimal disease and a consequent fall in tear volume and tear film thickness. This has been shown to be associated with a slowing of tear film lipid layer spreading (Yokoi et al. 2008), which could cause an increase in tear evaporation. This situation too would be negatively affected by a reduction in corneal sensitivity and a loss of sensory drive. In this case it is postulated that a functional EDE may be added to an organic ADDE, representing another hybrid combination.

> - Primary ADDE may lead to a secondary, functional EDE.
> - Primary EDE may lead to a secondary, functional ADDE.
> - Therefore, patients with moderate to severe dry eye will often have features of both ADDE and EDE, and it may be difficult to determine the primary cause.

The above proposals may explain why a clear clinical separation between ADDE and EDE may at times be difficult to support on the basis of substantive tests. Thus, while a decreased evaporation rate has been reported in ADDE by some authors (Hamano and Mitsunaga 1980; Tsubota and Yamada 1992; Goto et al. 2003), others, counter-intuitively, have reported an increase (Rolando et al. 1983; Mathers and Daley 1996) or have reported a marked overlap in values.

1.5.4 Other Complex Forms of Dry Eye

In addition to the hybrid dry eye forms described above, it is important to recognise that certain aetiologies of dry eye involve multiple mechanisms, with features of both ADDE and EDE or with symptoms arising from sources that are additional to or precede those arising from the dry eye itself. These include VKC and AKC, GVHD and Graves' disease and the symptoms of topical preservative toxicity.

MGD is a symptomatic disorder in its own right so that when it is of sufficient magnitude to give rise to evaporative dry eye, the symptoms of both MGD and dry eye may be combined. The symptoms of dry eye disease are well known and have been incorporated into numerous dry eye questionnaires, but there has been little attempt to distinguish those that might arise from the lids in MGD-related dry eye. Some possibilities that might be considered in future studies include redness of the lid margins in the absence of lash debris, itching of the lid margins and a need to rub the lids to obtain relief from symptoms. This omission is important in clinical trials, since treatment directed to the mechanisms of dry eye alone might fail to have an impact on symptoms arising from the lid margin due to MGD.

It is not uncommon, too, for MGD to occur in conjunction with anterior blepharitis so that their symptoms may be superimposed. They may both arise as a complication of systemic dermatoses such as rosacea, atopic dermatitis and seborrhoeic dermatitis (McCulley and Sciallis 1977; McCulley et al. 1982) and may be accompanied by an increased bacterial load as assessed by lid culture (Groden et al. 1991). Atopic dermatitis and use of systemic retinoids, in particular, have been associated with a high frequency of *S. aureus* culture (Seal and Pleyer 2007). There is evidence that commensal lid bacteria can influence Meibomian lipid composition and affect tear film lipid layer stability. *S. Aureus* growth can be stimulated by the presence of cholesterol, and in a study by Shine and McCulley (Shine et al. 1993), there were twice as many staphylococcal strains on the lid margins of those normal subjects whose Meibomian lipid was cholesterol rich than in the cholesterol-poor group. Normal lid commensals (coagulase-negative staphylococci [CoNS], *S. aureus* and *Propionibacterium acnes*) produce esterases and lipases which can release fatty acids and mono- and diglycerides into the tear film. These may be a source of irritation or of soap formation, said to be the basis of "Meibomian foam" (Dougherty and McCulley 1986).

Anterior Blepharitis and MGD

- Often occur together
- Can exacerbate each other
- Their symptoms may be superimposed

1.6   Summary

This chapter has provided a definition for dry eye disease that satisfies its major forms, aqueous-deficient and evaporative dry eye. Despite the clinical convenience of these groupings, evaporative water loss is the unifying aetiological factor in both sort of disease. Tear and ocular surface hyperosmolarity is the unifying mechanism. The many aetiological triggers and causes have been outlined here and form the framework for formulating diagnostic and therapeutic approaches.

Compliance with Ethical Requirements

Conflict of Interest Professor Bron declares the following relationships:

Diagnostear: Consultation

Redwood Pharma: Consultation

Santen: Consultation

TearLab: Advisory Board; ownership of stocks

Thea: Meeting travel and accommodation; honorarium

No animal or human studies were carried out by the author, for the preparation of this article.

References

Abelson MB, Holly FJ (1977) A tentative mechanism for inferior punctate keratopathy. Am J Ophthalmol 83:866–869

Alunno A, Carubbi F et al (2014) Unmasking the pathogenic role of IL-17 axis in primary Sjogren's syndrome: A new era for therapeutic targeting? Autoimmun Rev 51:38–43

Argüeso P, Balaram M et al (2002) Decreased levels of the goblet cell mucin MUC5AC in tears of patients with Sjogren syndrome. Invest Ophthalmol Vis Sci 43(4):1004–1011

Argüeso P, Tisdale A et al (2006) Mucin characteristics of human corneal-limbal epithelial cells that exclude the rose bengal anionic dye. Invest Ophthalmol Vis Sci 47(1):113–119

Argüeso P, Guzman-Aranguez A et al (2009) Association of cell surface mucins with galectin-3 contributes to the ocular surface epithelial barrier. J Biol Chem 284(34):23037–23045

Arita R, Itoh K et al (2008) Noncontact infrared meibography to document age-related changes of the meibomian glands in a normal population. Ophthalmology 115(5):911–915

Arita R, Itoh K et al (2010) Efficacy of diagnostic criteria for the differential diagnosis between obstructive meibomian gland dysfunction and aqueous deficiency dry eye. Jpn J Ophthalmol 54(5):387–391

Athappilly GK, Braverman RS (2009) Congenital alacrima in a patient with blepharophimosis syndrome. Ophthalmic Genet 30(1):37–39

Ban Y, Ogawa Y et al (2011) Morphologic evaluation of meibomian glands in chronic graft-versus-host disease using in vivo laser confocal microscopy. Mol Vis 17:2533–2543

Baudouin C (2001) The pathology of dry eye. Surv Ophthalmol Suppl 45:S211–S220

Baudouin C (2007) A new approach for better comprehension of diseases of the ocular surface. J Fr Ophtalmol 30(3):239–246

Baudouin C, Pisella PJ et al (1999) Dry eye syndromes and the ocular surface. J Fr Ophtalmol 22(8):893–902

Baudouin C, Labbe A et al (2010) Preservatives in eyedrops: the good, the bad and the ugly. Prog Retin Eye Res 29(4):312–334

Begley CG, Caffery B et al (2000) Responses of contact lens wearers to a dry eye survey. Optom Vis Sci 77(1):40–46

Begley CB, Chalmers RL et al (2001) Characterisation of ocular surface symptoms from optometric practices in North America. Cornea 20:610–618

Begley CG, Chalmers RL et al (2003) The relationship between habitual patient-reported symptoms and clinical signs among patients with dry eye of varying severity. Invest Ophthalmol Vis Sci 44(11):4753–4761

Benitez-Del-Castillo JM, Acosta MC et al (2007) Relation between corneal innervation with confocal microscopy and corneal sensitivity with noncontact esthesiometry in patients with dry eye. Invest Ophthalmol Vis Sci 48(1):173–181

Beuerman RW, Stern ME (2005) Neurogenic inflammation: a first line of defense for the ocular surface. Ocul Surf 3(4 Suppl):S203–S206

Blackie CA, Korb DR et al (2010) Nonobvious obstructive meibomian gland dysfunction. Cornea 29(12):1333–1345

Bourcier T, Acosta MC et al (2005) Decreased corneal sensitivity in patients with dry eye. Invest Ophthalmol Vis Sci 46(7):2341–2345

Brignole F, Pisella PJ et al (2000) Flow cytometric analysis of inflammatory markers in conjunctival epithelial cells of patients with dry eye. Invest Ophthalmol Vis Sci 41:1356–1363

Bron AJ, Argüeso P et al (2015) Clinical staining of the ocular surface-mechanisms and interpretations. Prog Retin Eye Res 44(1):36–61

Bron AJ, Tiffany JM (2004) The contribution of meibomian disease to dry eye. Ocul Surf 2(2):149–165

Bron AJ, Benjamin L et al (1991) Meibomian gland disease. Classification and grading of lid changes. Eye (Lond) 5(Pt 4):395–411

Bron AJ, Tiffany JM et al (2004) Functional aspects of the tear film lipid layer. Exp Eye Res 78(3):347–360

Bron AJ, Yokoi N et al (2009) Predicted phenotypes of dry eye: proposed consequences of its natural history. Ocul Surf 7(2):78–92

Brooks BP, Kleta R et al (2005) Genotypic heterogeneity and clinical phenotype in triple A syndrome: a review of the NIH experience 2000–2005. Clin Genet 68(3):215–221

Cedarstaff TH, Tomlinson A (1983) A comparative study of tear evaporation rates and water content of soft contact lenses. Am J Optom Physiol Opt 60(3):167–174

Chen HT, Chen KH et al (2004) Toxic keratopathy associated with abuse of low-dose anesthetic: a case report. Cornea 23(5):527–529

Chew CK, Jansweijer C et al (1993) An instrument for quantifying meibomian lipid on the lid margin: the Meibometer. Curr Eye Res 12(3):247–254

Collins MJ, Iskander DR et al (2006) Blinking patterns and corneal staining. Eye Contact Lens 32(6):287–293

Connor CG, Campbell JB et al (1994) The effects of daily wear contact lenses on goblet cell density. J Am Optom Assoc 65(11):792–794

Connor CG, Campbell JB et al (1997) The effects of disposable daily wear contact lenses on goblet cell count. CLAO J 23(1):37–39

Cope C, Dilly PN et al (1986) Wettability of the corneal surface: a reappraisal. Curr Eye Res 5:777–785

Craig JP, Tomlinson A (1997) Importance of the lipid layer in human tear film stability and evaporation. Optom Vis Sci 74(1):8–13

Dartt DA (2002) Regulation of mucin and fluid secretion by conjunctival epithelial cells. Prog Retin Eye Res 21(6):555–576

Dawson LJ, Stanbury J et al (2006) Antimuscarinic antibodies in primary Sjogren's syndrome reversibly inhibit the mechanism of fluid secretion by human submandibular salivary acinar cells. Arthritis Rheum 54(4):1165–1173

De Paiva CS, Pflugfelder SC (2004) Corneal epitheliopathy of dry eye induces hyperesthesia to mechanical air jet stimulation. Am J Ophthalmol 137(1):109–115

De Paiva CS, Corrales RM et al (2006) Corticosteroid and doxycycline suppress MMP-9 and inflammatory cytokine expression, MAPK activation in the corneal epithelium in experimental dry eye. Exp Eye Res 83(3):526–535

DEWS (2007a) The definition and classification of dry eye disease: report of the Definition and Classification Subcommittee of the International Dry Eye WorkShop (2007). Ocul Surf 5(2):75–92

DEWS (2007b) The epidemiology of dry eye disease: report of the Epidemiology Subcommittee of the International Dry Eye WorkShop (2007). Ocul Surf 5(2):93–107

Di Pascuale MA, Espana EM et al (2004) Clinical characteristics of conjunctivochalasis with or without aqueous tear deficiency. Br J Ophthalmol 88(3):388–392

Dougherty JM, McCulley JP (1986) Bacterial lipases and chronic blepharitis. Invest Ophthalmol Vis Sci 27:486–491

Doughty M, Fonn D et al (1997) A patient questionnaire approach to estimating the prevalence of dry eye symptoms in patients presenting to optometric practices across Canada. Optom Vis Sci 74:624–631

Efron N, Brennan N (1988) A survey of wearers of low water content hydrogel contact lenses. Clin Exp Optom 71:86–90

Fonn D, Situ P et al (1999) Hydrogel lens dehydration and subjective comfort and dryness ratings in symptomatic and asymptomatic contact lens wearers. Optom Vis Sci 76(10):700–704

Fortes MB, Diment BC et al (2011) Tear fluid osmolarity as a potential marker of hydration status. Med Sci Sports Exerc 43(8):1590–1597

Foulks G, Bron AJ (2003) A clinical description of meibomian gland dysfunction. Ocul Surf 1:107–126

Foulks GN, Borchman D et al (2010) Topical azithromycin therapy for meibomian gland dysfunction: clinical response and lipid alterations. Cornea 29(7):781–788

Fraunfelder FT, LaBraico JM et al (1985) Adverse ocular reactions possibly associated with isotretinoin. Am J Ophthalmol 100:534–537

Fraunfelder FT, Sciubba JJ et al (2012) The role of medications in causing dry eye. J Ophthalmol 2012:285851

Fu YA (1984) Ocular manifestation of polychlorinated biphenyls intoxication. Am J Ind Med 5(1–2):127–132

Gilbard JP, Farris RL (1983) Ocular surface drying and tear film osmolarity in thyroid eye disease. Acta Ophthalmol (Copenh) 61(1):108–116

Gipson IK, Hori Y et al (2004) Character of ocular surface mucins and their alteration in dry eye disease. Ocul Surf 2(2):131–148

Glasson MJ, Stapleton F et al (2003) Differences in clinical parameters and tear film of tolerant and intolerant contact lens wearers. Invest Ophthalmol Vis Sci 44(12):5116–5124

Gold-von Simson G, Axelrod FB (2006) Familial dysautonomia: update and recent advances. Curr Probl Pediatr Adolesc Health Care 36(6):218–237

Goto E, Tseng SC (2003) Differentiation of lipid tear deficiency dry eye by kinetic analysis of tear interference images. Arch Ophthalmol 121(2):173–180

Goto E, Endo K et al (2003) Tear evaporation dynamics in normal subjects and subjects with obstructive meibomian gland dysfunction. Invest Ophthalmol Vis Sci 44(2):533–539

Goto T, Zheng X et al (2004) Evaluation of the tear film stability after laser in situ keratomileusis using the tear film stability analysis system. Am J Ophthalmol 137(1):116–120

Groden LR, Murphy B et al (1991) Lid flora in blepharitis. Cornea 10(1):50–53

Hamano H, Mitsunaga S (1980) Application of an evaporimeter to the field of ophthalmology. J Jpn Cont Lens Soc 22:101–107

Hayashi Y, Arakaki R et al (2003) The role of caspase cascade on the development of primary Sjogren's syndrome. J Med Invest 50(1–2):32–38

Heath P (1949) Ocular lymphomas. Am J Ophthalmol 32(9):1213–1223

Hegab SM, al-Mutawa SA (1996) Congenital hereditary autosomal recessive alacrima. Ophthalmic Genet 17(1):35–38

Himebaugh NL, Begley CG et al (2009) Blinking and tear break-up during four visual tasks. Optom Vis Sci 86(2):E106–E114

Hori Y, Argueso P et al (2006) Mucins and contact lens wear. Cornea 25(2):176–181

Ibrahim OM, Matsumoto Y et al (2012) In vivo confocal microscopy evaluation of meibomian gland dysfunction in atopic-keratoconjunctivitis patients. Ophthalmology 119(10):1961–1968

Ishibashi T, Yokoi N et al (2003) Comparison of the short-term effects on the human corneal surface of topical timolol maleate with and without benzalkonium chloride. J Glaucoma 12(6):486–490

Itescu S, Brancato LJ et al (1990) A diffuse infiltrative CD8 lymphocytosis syndrome in human immunodeficiency virus (HIV) infection: a host immune response associated with HLA-DR5. Ann Intern Med 112:3–10

Iyer JV, Lee SY et al (2012) The dry eye disease activity log study. Scientific World Journal 2012:589875

Jaenen N, Baudouin C et al (2007) Ocular symptoms and signs with preserved and preservative-free glaucoma medications. Eur J Ophthalmol 17(3):341–349

James DG, Anderson R et al (1964) Ocular Sarcoidosis. Br J Ophthalmol 48:461–470

Jester JV, Nicolaides N et al (1989a) Meibomian gland dysfunction. I. Keratin protein expression in normal human and rabbit meibomian glands. Invest Ophthalmol Vis Sci 30:927–935

Jester JV, Nicolaides N et al (1989b) Meibomian gland dysfunction. II. The role of keratinization in a rabbit model of MGD. Invest Ophthalmol Vis Sci 30(5):936–945

Jordan A, Baum J (1980) Basic tear flow. Does it exist? Ophthalmology 87:920

Kim SH, Hwang S et al (2005) Two cases of lacrimal gland agenesis in the same family–clinicoradiologic findings and management. Can J Ophthalmol 40(4):502–505

King-Smith PE, Fink BA et al (2000) The thickness of the human precorneal tear film evidence from reflection spectra. Invest Ophthalmol Vis Sci 41:3348–3359

Knop E, Brewitt H (1992) Induction of conjunctival epithelial alterations by contact lens wearing. A prospective study. Ger J Ophthalmol 1(3–4):125–134

Knop E, Knop N et al (2011) The international workshop on meibomian gland dysfunction: report of the subcommittee on anatomy, physiology, and pathophysiology of the meibomian gland. Invest Ophthalmol Vis Sci 52(4):1938–1978

Korb DR, Herman JP et al (2005) Lid wiper epitheliopathy and dry eye symptoms. Eye Contact Lens 31(1):2–8

Korb DR, Herman JP et al (2010) Prevalence of lid wiper epitheliopathy in subjects with dry eye signs and symptoms. Cornea 29(4):377–383

Kunert KS, Keane-Myers AM et al (2001) Alteration in goblet cell numbers and mucin gene expression in a mouse model of allergic conjunctivitis. Invest Ophthalmol Vis Sci 42(11):2483–2489

Kunert KS, Tisdale AS et al (2002) Goblet cell numbers and epithelial proliferation in the conjunctiva of patients with dry eye syndrome treated with cyclosporine. Arch Ophthalmol 120(3):330–337

Kymionis GD, Plaka A et al (2011) Treatment of corneal dellen with a large diameter soft contact lens. Cont Lens Anterior Eye 34(6):290–292

Lemp MA (1995) Report of the National Eye Institute/Industry workshop on Clinical Trials in Dry Eyes. CLAO J 21(4):221–232

Lemp MA, Crews LA et al (2012) Distribution of aqueous-deficient and evaporative dry eye in a clinic-based patient cohort: a retrospective study. Cornea 31(5):472–478

Li DQ, Chen Z et al (2004) Stimulation of matrix metalloproteinases by hyperosmolarity via a JNK pathway in human corneal epithelial cells. Invest Ophthalmol Vis Sci 45(12):4302–4311

Lievens CW, Connor CG et al (2003) Comparing goblet cell densities in patients wearing disposable hydrogel contact lenses versus silicone hydrogel contact lenses in an extended-wear modality. Eye Contact Lens 29(4):241–244

Liu H, Begley C et al (2009) A link between tear instability and hyperosmolarity in dry eye. Invest Ophthalmol Vis Sci 50(8):3671–3679

Magalhaes M, Wenning GK et al (1995) Autonomic dysfunction in pathologically confirmed multiple system atrophy and idiopathic Parkinson's disease–a retrospective comparison. Acta Neurol Scand 91(2):98–102

Mathers WD (1993) Ocular evaporation in meibomian gland dysfunction and dry eye. Ophthalmology 100:347–351

Mathers WD, Daley TE (1996) Tear flow and evaporation in patients with and without dry eye. Ophthalmology 103(4):664–669

Mathers WD, Shields WJ et al (1991a) Meibomian gland morphology and tear osmolarity: changes with Accutane therapy. Cornea 10(4):286–290

Mathers WD, Shields WJ et al (1991b) Meibomian gland dysfunction in chronic blepharitis. Cornea 10(4):277–285

Mathers WD, Lane JA et al (1996) Model for ocular tear film function. Cornea 15(2):110–119

McCulley JP, Sciallis GF (1977) Meibomian keratoconjunctivitis. Am J Ophthalmol 84(6):788–793

McCulley JP, Dougherty JM et al (1982) Classification of chronic blepharitis. Ophthalmology 89(10):1173–1180

Moss SE, Klein R et al (2004) Incidence of dry eye in an older population. Arch Ophthalmol 122(3):369–373

Moss SE, Klein R et al (2008) Long-term incidence of dry eye in an older population. Optom Vis Sci 85(8):668–674

Nakamori K, Odawara M et al (1997) Blinking is controlled primarily by ocular surface conditions. Am J Ophthalmol 124:24–30

Nakamura H, Kawakami A et al (2006) Mechanisms of autoantibody production and the relationship between autoantibodies and the clinical manifestations in Sjogren's syndrome. Transl Res 148(6):281–288

Nelson JD, Shimazaki J et al (2011) The international workshop on meibomian gland dysfunction: report of the definition and classification subcommittee. Invest Ophthalmol Vis Sci 52(4):1930–1937

Nichols JJ, Sinnott LT (2006) Tear film, contact lens, and patient-related factors associated with contact lens-related dry eye. Invest Ophthalmol Vis Sci 47(4):1319–1328

Nichols KK, Nichols JJ et al (2004) The lack of association between signs and symptoms in patients with dry eye disease. Cornea 23(8):762–770

Nichols JJ, Ziegler C et al (2005) Self-reported dry eye disease across refractive modalities. Invest Ophthalmol Vis Sci 46(6):1911–1914

Nichols KK, Foulks GN et al (2011) The international workshop on meibomian gland dysfunction: executive summary. Invest Ophthalmol Vis Sci 52(4):1922–1929

Obata H (2006) Anatomy and histopathology of the human lacrimal gland. Cornea 25(10 Suppl 1):S82–S89

Ogawa Y, Kuwana M (2003) Dry eye as a major complication associated with chronic graft-versus-host disease after hematopoietic stem cell transplantation. Cornea 22(7 Suppl):S19–S27

Ogawa Y, Kuwana M et al (2003) Periductal area as the primary site for T-cell activation in lacrimal gland chronic graft-versus-host disease. Invest Ophthalmol Vis Sci 44(5):1888–1896

Ohnishi Y, Ikui S et al (1975) Further ophthalmic studies of patients with chronic chlorobiphenyls poisoning. Fukuoka Igaku Zasshi 66:640

Okun MS, Walter BL et al (2002) Beneficial effects of testosterone replacement for the nonmotor symptoms of Parkinson disease. Arch Neurol 59(11):1750–1753

Peng CC, Cerretani C et al (2014) Evaporation-driven instability of the precorneal tear film. Adv Colloid Interface Sci 206:250–264

Pharmakakis NM, Katsimpris JM et al (2002) Corneal complications following abuse of topical anesthetics. Eur J Ophthalmol 12(5):373–378

Pisella PJ, Malet F et al (2001) Ocular surface changes induced by contact lens wear. Cornea 20(8):820–825

Pisella PJ, Pouliquen P et al (2002) Prevalence of ocular symptoms and signs with preserved and preservative free glaucoma medication. Br J Ophthalmol 86(4):418–423

Pult H, Riede-Pult BH et al (2013) A new perspective on spontaneous blinks. Ophthalmology 120(5):1086–1091

Rees TD, Jelks GW (1981) Blepharoplasty and the dry eye syndrome: guidelines for surgery? Plast Reconstr Surg 68(2):249–252

Rolando M, Refojo MF et al (1983) Increased tear evaporation in eyes with keratoconjunctivitis sicca. Arch Ophthalmol 101:557–558

Rolando M, Brezzo G et al (1991) The effect o different benzalkonium chloride concentrations on human normal ocular surface. A controlled prospective impression cytology study. In: Lemp MA, Van Bijsterweld OP, Spinelli D (eds) The lacrimal system. Kugler & Ghedini, Amsterdam, pp 89–91

Rozsa AJ, Beuerman RW (1982) Density and organization of free nerve endings in the corneal epithelium of the rabbit. Pain 14(2):105–120

Sack RA, Beaton A et al (2000) Towards a closed eye model of the pre-ocular tear layer. Prog Retin Eye Res 19(6):649–668

Sarathi V, Shah NS (2010) Triple-A syndrome. Adv Exp Med Biol 685:1–8

Scherz W, Dohlman C (1975) Is the lacrimal gland dispensible? Keratoconjunctivitis sicca after lacrimal gland removal. Arch Ophthalmol 93:281–283

Schlanger JL (1993) A study of contact lens failures. J Am Optom Assoc 64(3):220–224

Seal D, Pleyer U (2007) Ocular infection. Informa Healthcare, New York

Seifert P, Spitznas M (1999) Vasoactive intestinal polypeptide (VIP) innervation of the human eyelid glands. Exp Eye Res 68(6):685–692

Shimazaki J, Sakata M et al (1995) Ocular surface changes and discomfort in patients with meibomian gland dysfunction. Arch Ophthalmol 113(10):1266–1270

Shimazaki J, Goto E et al (1998) Meibomian gland dysfunction in patients with Sjogren syndrome. Ophthalmology 105(8):1485–1488

Shine WE, Silvany R et al (1993) Relation of cholesterol-stimulated Staphylococcus aureus growth to chronic blepharitis. Invest Ophthalmol Vis Sci 34(7):2291–2296

Situ P, Simpson TL et al (2008) Conjunctival and corneal hyperesthesia in subjects with dryness symptoms. Optom Vis Sci 85(9):867–872

Slade SG, Linberg JV et al (1986) Control of lacrimal secretion after sphenopalatine ganglion block. Ophthal Plast Reconstr Surg 2(2):65–70

Sommer A, Emran N (1982) Tear production in a vitamin A responsive xerophthalmia. Am J Ophthalmol 93:84–87

Stern ME, Beuerman RW et al (1998) The pathology of dry eye: the interaction between the ocular surface and lacrimal glands. Cornea 17(6):584–589

Stern ME, Gao J et al (2004) The role of the lacrimal functional unit in the pathophysiology of dry eye. Exp Eye Res 78(3):409–416

Sullivan BD, Crews LA et al (2014) Correlations between commonly used objective signs and symptoms for the diagnosis of dry eye disease: clinical implications. Acta Ophthalmol 92(2):161–166

Tamura M, Murata N et al (2008) Facial nerve function insufficiency after radiosurgery versus microsurgery. Prog Neurol Surg 21:108–118

Tang NE, Zuure PL et al (2000) Reflex lacrimation in patients with glaucoma and healthy control subjects by fluorophotometry. Invest Ophthalmol Vis Sci 41(3):709–714

Tei M, Spurr-Michaud SJ et al (2000) Vitamin A deficiency alters the expression of mucin genes by the rat ocular surface epithelium. Invest Ophthalmol Vis Sci 41(1):82–88

Tiffany JM (1990a) Measurement of wettability of the corneal epithelium. 1. Particle attachment method. Acta Ophthalmol 68:175–181

Tiffany JM (1990b) Measurement of wettability of the corneal epithelium. 2. Contact angle method. Acta Ophthalmol 68:182–187

Tomlinson A, Khanal S (2005) Assessment of tear film dynamics: quantification approach. Ocul Surf 3(2):81–95

Tsubota K (1998) Tear dynamics and dry eye. Prog Retin Eye Res 17(4):565–596

Tsubota K, Nakamori K (1995) Effects of ocular surface area and blink rate on tear dynamics. Arch Ophthalmol 113(2):155–158

Tsubota K, Yamada M (1992) Tear evaporation from the ocular surface. Invest Ophthalmol Vis Sci 33(10):2942–2950

Tung CI, Perin AF et al (2014) Tear meniscus dimensions in tear dysfunction and their correlation with clinical parameters. Am J Ophthalmol 157(2):301–310 e301

Walsh NP, Fortes MB et al (2012) Is whole-body hydration an important consideration in dry eye? Invest Ophthalmol Vis Sci 53(10):6622–6627

Xu KP, Yagi Y et al (1996) Decrease in corneal sensitivity and change in tear function in dry eye. Cornea 15(3):235–239

Yeh S, Song XJ et al (2003) Apoptosis of ocular surface cells in experimentally induced dry eye. Invest Ophthalmol Vis Sci 44(1):124–129

Yokoi N, Takehisa Y et al (1996) Correlation of tear lipid layer interference patterns with the diagnosis and severity of dry eye. Am J Ophthalmol 122:818–824

Yokoi N, Mossa F et al (1999) Assessment of meibomian gland function in dry eye using meibometry. Arch Ophthalmol 117(6):723–729

Yokoi N, Komuro A et al (2005) Clinical impact of conjunctivochalasis on the ocular surface. Cornea 24(8 Suppl):S24–S31

Yokoi N, Yamada H et al (2008) Rheology of tear film lipid layer spread in normal and aqueous tear-deficient dry eyes. Invest Ophthalmol Vis Sci 49(12):5319–5324

Yokoi N, Bron AJ, et al (2014) The precorneal tear film as a fluid shell: the effect of blinking and saccades on tear film distribution and dynamics. Ocul Surf 12(4):252–266

Zhang X, Volpe EA et al (2012) NK cells promote Th-17 mediated corneal barrier disruption in dry eye. PLoS One 7(5):e36822

Zhao H-C, Jumblatt JE et al (2001) Quantification of MUC5AC protein in human tears. Cornea 20:873–877

Zoukhri D (2006) Effect of inflammation on lacrimal gland function. Exp Eye Res 82(5):885–898

The Epidemiology of Dry Eye Disease

2

Fiona Stapleton, Qian Garrett, Colin Chan, and Jennifer P. Craig

2.1 Impact of Dry Eye Disease

Dry eye disease (DED) is a common and chronic condition, which is considered a major health concern internationally. It causes eye discomfort and pain; it limits vision and reduces quality of life (Reddy et al. 2004). Those with dry eye are two to three times more likely to report problems with everyday activities such as reading, performing professional work, computer use, watching television, and daytime or nighttime driving (Schaumberg et al. 2003, 2009; Miljanovic et al. 2007). Dry eye disease also impacts socially, as those with dry eye and refractive errors are unsuitable for refractive surgery and are limited in their ability to wear contact lenses or use cosmetics (Reddy et al. 2004; Miljanovic et al. 2007).

F. Stapleton, BSc, MSc, PhD, MCOptom, FAAO, FBCLA, DCLP, GradCertOcTher (✉)
Q. Garrett, PhD
School of Optometry and Vision Science,
University of New South Wales,
Sydney, NSW, Australia
e-mail: f.stapleton@unsw.edu.au

C. Chan, MBBS (Hons) FRANZCO
Vision Eye Institute, School of Optometry and Vision Science, University of New South Wales,
270 Victoria Ave, Chatswood, Sydney,
NSW 2067, Australia
e-mail: colin.chan@visioneyeinstitute.com.au

J.P. Craig, PhD, MCOptom
Department of Ophthalmology, School of Optometry and Vision Sciences, University of Auckland,
Auckland, New Zealand

Dry eye may also compromise outcomes of cataract surgery.

> Those with dry eye are two to three times more likely to report problems with everyday activities such as reading, performing professional work, computer use, watching television, and daytime or nighttime driving.

Dry eye disease is a significant problem for up to 35 % of the population, and two-thirds of sufferers are women, with a higher risk in postmenopausal women (Chia et al. 2003). More severe dry eye affects 8 % of women and 4 % of men over 50 years of age (Schaumberg et al. 2003, 2009). Dry eye is the most commonly reported reason for seeking medical eye care, and thus dry eye has a significant cost due to direct and indirect healthcare costs and through reduced productivity at work (Moss et al. 2000). The economic burden of dry eye is substantial: in the United States, the average cost of dry eye management was estimated to be US\$ 11,302 per sufferer and US\$ 55 billion overall (Yu et al. 2011). The annual cost to treat dry eye including direct costs, such as oral and topical medication, punctal plugs, practitioner visits, and nutritional supplements and indirect costs, was \$783 (range \$757–\$809) or \$3.84 billion (Yu et al. 2011). Utility assessment studies suggest that severe dry eye disease impacts life to a similar extent as moderate to severe angina, and

C. Chan (ed.), *Dry Eye: A Practical Approach*, Essentials in Ophthalmology,
DOI 10.1007/978-3-662-44106-0_2, © Springer-Verlag Berlin Heidelberg 2015

in the most severe cases, the utility was poorer than for a hip fracture (Schiffman et al. 2003; Bushholz et al. 2006). Dry eye disease comprises approximately 20 % of presentations to hospital outpatient clinics (Hikichi et al. 1995; Onwubiko et al. 2014) and 11–20 % of presentations to optometric practice (Doughty et al. 1997; Albietz 2000).

> - Dry eye is the most common reason for seeking eye care.
> - Dry eye is more common in women, and women are more likely than men to suffer from severe dry eye.

Dry eye is poorly controlled with current therapy; hence, those with severe disease suffer chronically with symptoms for over 200 days each year and exhaust on average 50 % of their annual sick leave due to dry eye (Schiffman et al. 2003). Less severe (non-Sjögrens) disease interferes with work for 191 days per year and resulted in 2 days of absenteeism per year (Nelson et al. 2000). There have been limited studies to evaluate the impact of therapies on long-term patient-reported outcomes or their economic impact. With increased life expectancy and an aging population, the economic and social impacts of this condition would be expected to grow substantially.

> - Current treatment for dry eye is inadequate resulting in ongoing symptoms and repeat eye-care visits.
> - An aging population will only increase the economic burden of dry eye.

There have been significant advances in our understanding of the epidemiology of DED over the past 10 years largely due to a better understanding of the underlying causes of the condition, namely, tear osmolarity and ocular surface inflammation. The 2007 International Dry Eye Workshop of the Tear Film and Ocular Surface Society defined DED as "a multifactoral disease of the tears and ocular surface that results in symptoms of discomfort, visual disturbance and tear film instability with potential damage to the ocular surface. It is accompanied by increased osmolarity of the tear film and inflammation of the ocular surface" (2007).

Dry eye disease occurs when the tear film is compromised by reduced aqueous tear production and/or excessive tear evaporation, and the disease can be broadly classified as either aqueous deficient or evaporative, although practically subjects with dry eye disease frequently manifest with signs consistent with both classifications, and the subtypes are not exclusive. Evaporative dry eye due to meibomian gland dysfunction appears to represent the most common DED subtype in both population and outpatient clinic cohorts (Tong et al. 2010; Lemp et al. 2012; Viso et al. 2012), where 45–65 % of those with dry eye symptoms have MGD, although many with MGD lack dry eye symptoms. This chapter will summarize the frequency of disease and relevant risk factors for both classes of dry eye disease where possible.

> Meibomian gland dysfunction (MGD) is the most common subtype of dry eye disease.

2.2 Prevalence of Dry Eye Disease

Early reports of the prevalence of DED showed markedly variable results partly due to the different disease definitions used in these studies and the lack of a single validated test or combination of tests to confirm a diagnosis. The Epidemiology Subcommittee of the 2007 DEWS reviewed major epidemiological studies of dry eye and demonstrated that the prevalence of dry eye ranged from 5 to 30 % of individuals aged over 50 (2007). Their consensus was that the prevalence of severe disease was likely to be at the low end of this range and that the true prevalence of mild or episodic disease was closer to the upper end of this range. Higher rates are generally observed with questionnaire-based studies and in clinic-based studies, with lower rates amongst intention to treat or treatment studies.

> - Prevalence estimates of dry eye disease range from 5 to 30 % of people over the age of 50.
> - Prevalence estimates vary because of nonstandardized definitions.
> - A large proportion of individuals with dry eye disease are asymptomatic.

Prevalence estimates of DED both from key population-based and records analyses are shown in Table 2.1. The recent findings are broadly consistent with those reported in the DEWS report from 2007, with higher rates associated with age and gender. Compared with recent studies in Caucasian populations (USA Beaver Dam Study, Beaver Dam Offspring Study, Physicians Health Study, Veterans Affairs Database Audit), those in Asian populations (Korea, China – Beijing Eye Study and Japan) showed a consistently higher prevalence, following adjustment for age and gender. Based on the body of evidence, it would be appropriate to consider race as a confirmed risk factor for DED.

Prevalence estimates of MGD have been similarly confounded by the lack of a standardized definition and standardized method for grading MGD (Schaumberg et al. 2011). There are also no standardized questionnaires available for MGD; symptoms frequently overlap with those reported in dry eye disease and/or anterior blepharitis, and the disease is frequently asymptomatic (Viso et al. 2012). Estimates of prevalence from population-based studies have varied widely from 3.5 to 68.3 % (Schein et al. 1997; Jie et al. 2008; Siak et al. 2012).

Table 2.2 summarizes the key population studies and their disease definitions. Key features are firstly that lower prevalence rates have been published in studies where symptoms were not included as part of the disease definition. The clinical signs used as part of the diagnostic criteria have also varied widely, with some studies focusing on secondary outcomes such as measures of tear quality or tear stability and others on specific but varied lid signs. The relatively high prevalence rate of 68 % from the Beijing Eye Study, for example, is consistent with a definition that included clinical signs of lid disease and symptoms of dry eye. Secondly, the prevalence data appears to be consistently higher in studies of Asian populations compared with reports where the majority of participants are Caucasian for broadly similar disease definitions and sampling techniques (Schein et al. 1997; Lin et al. 2003; Uchino et al. 2011; Siak et al. 2012; Viso et al. 2012).

> - Meibomian gland dysfunction appears to be more common in Asian populations.
> - The prevalence of meibomian gland dysfunction is likely to increase with age and to be higher in the female population.

There have been few age-specific prevalence studies on MGD. There is limited consensus on the impact of age on MGD with Asian studies showing no impact of age. These generally confirm that MGD is the more common subtype and demonstrate a 2.5× higher rate of asymptomatic MGD compared to a Caucasian population.

However, it would be logical if dry eye disease prevalence increases with age, that MGD as the most common subtype of dry eye disease would most likely increase in prevalence with age. One Spanish study (Viso et al. 2012) looked at both asymptomatic and symptomatic MGD in over a thousand patients over 40. This study found that both asymptomatic and symptomatic MGD prevalence increased with age. The same study found that asymptomatic but not symptomatic MGD was more common in males than females. Again like age, very few gender-specific prevalence studies have been done on MGD. Overall most studies seem to point that dry eye disease is more common in women and that women are more at risk of severe dry eye disease. Again logically, since MGD is the most common subtype of dry eye disease, it could be expected that prevalence and severity of MGD should be higher in women.

Table 2.1 Prevalence of all dry eyes (large cohort studies or records analyses)

Authors	Study duration	Region/country	Population studied	Age (years)	Definition	Denominator	Prevalence	95 % CI
Schein et al. (1997)	1993–1995	USA	2,420 participants in the Salisbury Eye Study	65≤	At least one (of six) symptoms occurring often or always	2,420	14.6 %	13.2–16.0 %
McCarty et al. (1998)		Australia	926 participants in the Melbourne Visual Impairment project. 493 females, 433 males	40≤	At least one (of six) symptoms (not attributed to hay fever) rated as severe	926	Symptoms 5.5 % 1.5–16.3 % objective tests	4.0–7.0 %
Moss et al. (2000)	1995–2005	USA	3,722 participants in the 5- and 10- year Beaver Dam Eye Study	63±10 (48–91)	Self-report to questions "For the past 3 months or longer have you had dry eyes?"	2,414 (44 % men)	All subjects 21.6 % 48–59 17.3 % 80<28.0 %* Men 17.2 % Women 25.0 %*	19.9–23.3 %
Chia et al. (2003)	1999–2001	Australia	1,174 participants in the Blue Mountains Eye Study	60.8 (50–90)	At least one (of 4) symptoms, regardless of severity or at least 1 symptom rated either moderate or severe	1,075	16.6 % (at least one symptom) 15.3 % (3 or more symptoms)	14.3–18.7 % 13.1–17.5 %
Schaumberg et al. (2003)	1992–1996	USA	38,124 female participants in Women's Health Study	49–89	History of clinically diagnosed DED or severe symptoms constantly or often	36,995	7.8 % (age adjusted prevalence for women over 50)	7.5–8.1 %
Schaumberg et al. (2009)	1997–2004	USA	25,444 men, participants in Physicians Health Studies I or II	64.3 (50–90)	Clinically diagnosed dry eye or severe symptoms (both dryness and irritation constantly or often)	25,444	Men 4.3 % 50–54 3.9 % 80<7.7 %*	4.1–4.5 % 3.7–4.1 %
Galor et al. (2011)	2005–2010	USA	Data extracted from the Miami and Broward Veterans Affairs database. Total 16,862	21–90	International Classification of Disease, 9th edition, Clinical Modification (ICD-9-CM) code 375.15	16,862	All subjects 10 % Male 12 % Female 22 %	9.5–10.5 %
Viso et al. (2012)	2005–2006	Spain	1,155 from National Health Service Registry	63.6±14.4 (40–96)	Symptoms and at least one of Schirmer test score ≤5 mm, TBUT ≤10 s, fluorescein staining score ≥1, and rose bengal score ≥3	654 (32.7 % 243 males, 411 females 62.8 %)	All subjects 11 %	8.6–13.3 %
Paulsen et al. (2014)	2005–2008	USA	3,275 Beaver Dam Offspring Study (BOSS) participants. 1,789 females (54.9%)	21–84	Self-report of frequency and the intensity of symptoms and use of eyedrops at least once a day	3,275	14.5 % Men 10.5 % Women 17.9 %	13.3–15.7 %

Lee et al. (2002)	2001	Indonesia	1,058 selected from 100 households, predominantly rural population	21≤	At least one (of six) symptoms often or all of the time	1,058	Age adjusted rate 27.5 %	24.8–30.2 %
							21–29 19.2 %	15.0–23.5 %
							60<30.0 %	20.1–39.5 %
Lin et al. (2003)	1999–2000	Taiwan	2,038 participants in the Shihpai Eye Study	65≤	At least one (of 6) symptoms often or all of the time	1,361	33.7 %	32.4–34.9 %
Han et al. (2011)	2008–2009	Korea	657 (317 males (48.2%), 340 female (51.8%)). 346 urban and 311 rural participants	72 (65–95)	One + symptoms of dry eye often or most of the time, and at least one of: TBUT ≤10 s, Schirmer score ≤5 mm, and corneal staining ≥ grade 1	657	Age, gender, rural adjusted 33.2 %	28.8–37.3 %
Jie et al. (2009)	2001	Beijing, China	4,439 previous participants in the Beijing Eye study 2001	57 (40–84)	One + of the following: TBUT ≤10 s; Schirmer ≤5 mm; fluorescein staining ≥1, lid margin telangiectasia; and/or plugging of the gland orifices. OR TBUT ≤4 s or Schirmer ≤4 mm, or fluorescein staining ≥2	1,957 (1,112 females)	21 %	19.2–22.8 %
Zhang et al. (2012)	2010	Shandong, China	1,902 senior high school students		Either a previous diagnosis of DES or severe symptoms (both dryness and irritation constantly or often) per Schaumberg et al. (2003)	1,885 (958 male, 927 female)	23.7 %	21.8–25.6 %
Guo et al. (2010)	Jun–Sep 2006	Mongolia	2,112 native Mongolians (1,125 male (53.3%))	54.9±11.7 (40–91)	One or more symptoms often or all the time	1,816	50.1 %	47.8–52.4 %
Uchino et al. (2011)	Feb – Mar 2010	Japan	3,294	40–≥80	Severe symptoms of DED (both ocular dryness and irritation either constantly or often or clinically diagnosed DED as reported by participants	2,644 (1,211 men and 1,423 women)	21.6 % women	19.5–23.9 %
							12.5 % men	10.7–14.5 %
Uchino et al. (2013)		Japan	561 Japanese young and middle aged office workers using VDTs	22–65	One or more symptoms of dry eye often or most of the time, and at least one of: TBUT ≤10 s, Schirmer ≤5 mm, and fluorescein staining ≥ grade 1	561 Office (187 women, 374 men)	18.7 % (women)	13.4–25.1 %
							8.0 % (men)	5.5–11.3 %

Shaded studies represent those carried out in Asian populations

TBUT tear breakup time

*Statistically significant effect of age or gender

Table 2.2 Prevalence of evaporative dry eye

Authors	Study duration	Region/country	Population studied	Age range	Definition	Denominator	Prevalence	95 % CI
Viso et al. (2009)	May 2005–Mar 2006	Spain	1,155 from National Health Service Registry,	63.6 ± 14.4 (40–96)	Viscous or waxy secretion or no secretion at all upon digital expression, lid margin telangiectasia, or plugging of the gland orifices	654 (32.7 % 243 males, 411 females 62.8 %)	30.5 % In those with dry eye 45.8 %	26.9–34.1 % 34.8–57.2 %
Viso et al. (2012)	May 2005 – Mar 2006	Spain	619. 229 males (37 %) and 390 females (63 %)	63.4 (40–96)	One or more of: (1) absent, viscous or waxy white secretion upon digital expression; (2) presence of two or more lid margin telangiectases; and (3) plugging of two or more gland orifices	619	Asymptomatic MGD 21.9 % Symptomatic MGD 8.6 %	18.8–25.3 % 6.7–10.9 %
Siak et al. (2012)		Singapore	3,271 (51.8 % females) in the Singapore Malay eye study (SiMES)	40–79	Either lid margin telangiectasia or gland orifice plugging in at least one eye	3,271	56.3%	53.3–59.4 %
Lin et al. (2003)	1999–2000	Taiwan	2,038 participants in the Shihpai Eye Study	65≤	Telangiectasia at the lid margin or plugging of the gland orifices	1,361	60.8%	59.5–62.1 %
Molinari et al. (2000)	1999	USA	226 (113 active duty forces (ADF), 113 US veterans (USV))	23.2 for ADF 68.1 years for USV	Signs of inability to express; not clear, mildly turbid; mild hyperemia; exclusion cysts over meibomian gland orifices but with no symptoms only with mild irritation	113 ADF; 113 US USV	5.3 % MGD in ADF (all CL wearers) 14.2 % MGD in USV (non CL wearers)	1.7–9.4 % 7.8–20.6 %
Home et al. (1990)		USA	398	10–60≤	Cloudy or absent gland secretion upon repeated expression of the lower lid	398 (200 males, 198 females)	38.9 % 10–19; 18.2 % 20–29; 33.3 % 30–39; 40 % 40–49; 34.9 % 50–59; 51.4 % >60; 67.2 %	34.1–43.7

Table 2.3 Risk factors for dry eye

Level of evidence		
Mostly consistent[a]	Suggestive[b]	Unclear[c]
Older age	Asian race	Cigarette smoking
Female sex	Medications	Hispanic ethnicity
Postmenopausal estrogen therapy	Tricyclic antidepressants	
Omega-3 and omega-6 fatty acids	Selective serotonin reuptake inhibitors	Anticholinergics
Medications	Diuretics	Anxiolytics
Antihistamines	Beta-blockers	Antipsychotics
Connective tissue disease	Diabetes mellitus	Alcohol
LASIK and refractive excimer laser surgery	HIV/HTLV1 infection	Menopause
Radiation therapy	Systemic chemotherapy	Botulinum toxin injection
Hematopoietic stem cell transplantation	Large incision ECCE and penetrating keratoplasty	
	Isotretinoin	Acne
Vitamin A deficiency	Low humidity environments	Gout
Hepatitis C infection	Sarcoidosis	Oral contraceptives
Androgen deficiency	Ovarian dysfunction	Pregnancy

Reprinted the epidemiology of dry eye disease: report of the Epidemiology Subcommittee of The International Dry Eye Workshop (2007) with permission from Elsevier)

[a]Mostly consistent evidence implies the existence of at least one adequately powered and otherwise well-conducted study published in a peer-reviewed journal, along with the existence of a plausible biological rationale and corroborating basic research or clinical data

[b]Suggestive evidence implies the existence of either (1) inconclusive information from peer-reviewed publications or (2) inconclusive or limited information to support the association, but either not published or published somewhere other than in a peer-reviewed journal

[c]Unclear evidence implies either directly conflicting information in peer-reviewed publications or inconclusive information but with some basis for biological rationale

2.3   Risk Factors for Dry Eye Disease

Higher prevalence rates are consistently reported with:

1. Age
2. Female gender, estrogen therapy in postmenopausal women, and androgen deficiency

   The meibomian glands are thought to be partially under hormonal influence with androgen/estrogen balance affecting function. A relative lack of androgen or relative excess of estrogen is thought to promote meibomian gland dysfunction.

3. Systemic antihistamines
4. LASIK and refractive surgery

   Dry eye is a recognized complication due to refractive surgery. Disruption of the corneal sensory nerves leads to a relative neuro-trophia and disruption of the normal lacrimal reflex arc.

5. Radiation therapy
6. Vitamin A deficiency
7. Hepatitis C infection
8. Hematopoietic stem cell transplantation

   Ocular graft-versus-host disease can occur in patients after bone marrow transplantation.

A range of other risk factors with varying levels of evidence was proposed by this review (Table 2.3). Environmental factors not mentioned in Table 2.1 but frequently associated with dry eye are contact lens wear and computer/visual display terminal use. A significant proportion of contact lens wearers (50–75 %) experience dry eye symptoms, and this is a major reason for discontinuation of contact lens wear. Computer use may cause dry eye symptoms due to prolonged visual attention and an associated reduced blink rate.

2.4 Summary

The prevalence of dry eye disease may be as high as 33 % in some populations, with moderate to severe disease affecting 5–10 % of individuals. The frequency of DED varies considerably with diagnostic criteria for DED although there is concordance in the major risk factors identified from well-designed population studies. There are clearly significant societal costs associated with this major public health concern, particularly given the disease chronicity and limited management options, and these costs will escalate in the future with an aging population. Future directions will include the development of rational treatments based on better understanding of the disease pathophysiology and the design of studies to elucidate the impact of therapy on the economic costs of disease. Population-based studies should employ standardized classification criteria and outcome measures including biomarkers to better elucidate the epidemiology and natural history of different subtypes of dry eye.

Compliance with Ethical Requirements Fiona Stapleton, Qian Garrett, and Jennifer Craig declare that they have no conflict of interest. No human or animal studies were carried out by the authors for this article.

References

Albietz J (2000) Prevalence of dry eye subtypes in clinical optometry practice. Optom Vis Sci 77:357–363

Bushholz P, Steeds CS, Stern LS et al (2006) Utility assessment to measure the impact of dry eye disease. Ocul Surf 4:155–161

Chia E-M, Mitchell P, Rochtchina E, Lee AJ, Maroun R, Wang JJ (2003) Prevalence and associations of dry eye syndrome in an older population: the Blue Mountains Eye Study. Clin Experiment Ophthalmol 31(3): 229–232

Doughty MJ, Fonn D, Richter D, Simpson T, Caffery B, Gordon K (1997) A patient questionnaire approach to estimating the prevalence of dry eye symptoms in patients presenting to optometric practices across Canada. Optom Vis Sci 74:624–631

Galor A, Feuer W, Lee DJ, Florez H, Carter D, Pouyeh B, Prunty WJ, Perez VL (2011) Prevalence and risk factors of dry eye syndrome in a United States Veterans Affairs population. Am J Ophthalmol 152(3):377. e372–384.e372

Guo B, Lu P, Chen X, Zhang W, Chen R (2010) Prevalence of dry eye disease in Mongolians at high altitude in China: the henan eye study. Ophthalmic Epidemiol 17(4):234–241

Han S, Hyon J, Woo S, Lee J, Kim T, Kim K (2011) Prevalence of dry eye disease in an elderly Korean population. Arch Ophthalmol 129(5):633–638

Hikichi T, Yoshida A, Fukui Y, Hamano T, Ri M, Araki K, Horimoto K, Takamura E, Kitagawa K, Oyama M (1995) The epidemiology of dry eye in Japanese eye centres. Graefes Arch Clin Exp Ophthalmol 233: 995–998

Jie Y, Xu L, Wu YY, Jonas JB (2008) Prevalence of dry eye among adult Chinese in the Beijing Eye Study. Eye (Lond) 23(3):688–693

Jie Y, Xu L, Wu YY, Jonas JB. Prevalence of dry eye among adult Chinese in the Beijing Eye Study (2009) Eye 23:688–693

Lee AJ, Lee J, Saw S-M, Gazzard G, Koh D, Widjaja D, Tan DTH (2002) Prevalence and risk factors associated with dry eye symptoms: a population based study in Indonesia. Br J Ophthalmol 86(12):1347–1351

Lemp MA, Crews LA, Bron AJ, Foulks GN, Sullivan BD (2012) Distribution of aqueous-deficient and evaporative dry eye in a clinic-based patient cohort: a retrospective study. Cornea 31(5):472–478

Lin PY, Tsai SY, Cheng CY, Liu JH, Chou P, Hsu WM (2003) Prevalence of dry eye among an elderly Chinese population in Taiwan: The Shihpai Eye Study. Ophthalmology 110:109–1101

McCarty CA, Bansal AK, Livingston PM, Stanislavsky YL, Taylor HR (1998) The epidemiology of dry eye in Melbourne, Australia. Ophthalmology 105:1114–1119

Miljanovic B, Dana R, Sullivan DA, Schaumberg DA (2007) Impact of dry eye syndrome on vision-related quality of life. Am J Ophthalmol 143(3):409.e402–415.e402

Moss SE, Klein R, Klein BE (2000) Prevalence of and risk factors for dry eye syndrome. Arch Ophthalmol 118(9):1264–1268

Nelson JD, Helms H, Fiscella R, Southwell Y, Hirsch JD (2000) A new look at dry eye disease and its treatment. Adv Ther 17(2):84–93

Onwubiko SN, Eze BI, Udeh NN, Arinze OC, Onwasigwe EN, Umeh RE (2014) Dry eye disease: prevalence, distribution and determinants in a hospital-based population. Cont Lens Anterior Eye 37(3):157–161

Paulsen AJ, Cruickshanks KJ, Fischer ME, Huang G-H, Klein BEK, Klein R, Dalton DS (2014) Dry eye in the beaver dam offspring study: prevalence, risk factors, and health-related quality of life. Am J Ophthalmol 157(4):799–806

Reddy P, Grad O, Rajagopalan K (2004) The economic burden of dry eye: a conceptual framework and preliminary assessment. Cornea 23(8):751

Schaumberg DA, Sullivan DA, Buring JE, Dana R (2003) Prevalence of dry eye syndrome among US women. Am J Ophthalmol 136:318–326

Schaumberg DA, Dana R, Buring JE, Sullivan DA (2009) Prevalence of dry eye disease among us men: estimates from the physicians' health studies. Arch Ophthalmol 127(6):763–768

Schaumberg DA, Nichols JJ, Papas EB, Tong L, Uchino M, Nichols KK (2011) The international workshop on meibomian gland dysfunction: report of the subcommittee on the epidemiology of, and associated risk factors for, MGD. Invest Ophthalmol Vis Sci 52(4):1994–2005

Schein OD, Munoz B, Tielsch JM, Bandeen-Roche K, West SK (1997) Prevalence of dry eye among the elderly. Am J Ophthalmol 124(6):723–728

Schiffman RM, Walt JG, Jacobsen G, Doyle JJ, Lebovics G, Sumner W (2003) Utility assessment among patients with dry eye disease. Ophthalmology 110(7): 1412–1419

Siak JJK, Tong L, Wong WL, Cajucom-Uy H, Rosman M, Saw SM, Wong TY (2012) Prevalence and risk factors of meibomian gland dysfunction: the Singapore Malay eye Study. Cornea 31:1223–1228

The definition and classification of dry eye disease: report of the Definition and Classification Subcommittee of the International Dry Eye Workshop (2007) Ocul Surf 5(2):75–92

The Epidemiology of dry eye disease: report of the Epidemiology Subcommittee of the International Dry Eye Workshop (2007) Ocul Surf 5(2):93–107

Tong L, Chaurasia SS, Mehta JS, Beuerman RW (2010) Screening for meibomian gland disease: its relation to dry eye subtypes and symptoms in a tertiary referral clinic in Singapore. Invest Ophthalmol Vis Sci 51(7):3449–3454

Uchino M, Nishiwaki Y, Michikawa T, Shirakawa K, Kuwahara E, Yamada M, Dogru M, Schaumberg DA, Kawakita T, Takebayashi T, Tsubota K (2011) Prevalence and risk factors of dry eye disease in Japan: Koumi study. Ophthalmology 118(12):2361–2367. doi:10.1016/j.ophtha.2011.05.029, Epub 2011 Sep 1

Uchino M, Yokoi N, Uchino Y, et al. Prevalence of dry eye disease and its risk factors in visual display terminal users: the Osaka study (2013) Am J Ophthalmol 156:759–766

Viso E, Rodriguez-Ares MT, Gude F (2009) Prevalence of and associated factors for dry eye in a Spanish adult population (the Salnes Eye Study). Ophthalmic Epidemiol 16(1):15–21

Viso E, Rodríguez-Ares MT, Abelenda D, Oubiña B, Gude F (2012) Prevalence of asymptomatic and symptomatic meibomian gland dysfunction in the general population of Spain. Invest Ophthalmol Vis Sci 53(6):2601–2606. doi:10.1167/iovs.11-9228

Yu J, Asche CV, Fairchild CJ (2011) The economic burden of dry eye disease in the United States: a decision tree analysis. Cornea 30:379–387

Zhang Y, Chen H, Wu X (2012) Prevalence and risk factors associated with dry eye syndrome among senior high school students in a county of shandong province, china. Ophthalmic Epidemiol 19(4):226–230

Practical Office-Based Screening and Diagnostics

Colin Chan

It is vital to have a standard routine screening and diagnostic protocol for dry eye in the clinic. This is essential because:

1. Dry eye visits account for a significant proportion of new and repeat consultations (Yu et al. 2011; Reddy et al. 2004).
2. Dry eye consults can be time consuming.
3. Dry eye can affect patient satisfaction especially post cataract and refractive surgery (Woodward et al. 2009; Levinson et al. 2008; Solomon et al. 2009; Nettune and Pflugfelder 2010; Gayton 2009).

25 % of patients who visit ophthalmic clinics report symptoms of dry eye.

The meibomian gland dysfunction workshop produced by TFOS (Tear Film and Ocular Surface Society) has recommendations for what should be used routinely as diagnostic tests for dry eye (Table 3.1) (Nichols et al. 2011). These tests are obviously beyond the means for most ophthalmologists and optometrists in terms of time and equipment. It is also well beyond what is done in current routine practice (Downie et al. 2013).

A practical approach to diagnosis needs to be more abbreviated and selective. The order that tests are performed is also important. The performance of one test needs to ideally not affect the result of the next.

For example, Schirmer testing will cause significant irritation and inferior punctate epithelial erosions. This obviously will affect the examination findings with fluorescein.

My suggested order of tests would be (Nichols et al. 2011):

1. Symptom questionnaire
2. Clinical history
3. Tear film break-up time (TFBUT) with fluorescein
4. Corneal staining with fluorescein
5. Schirmer 1
6. Lid margin examination
7. Meibomian gland expression

3.1 Focusing Your Diagnostic Testing

The focus of your diagnostic testing should be to identify a few key questions necessary to guide management.

Table 3.2 summarizes current diagnostic methods that can achieve this effectively and efficiently.

C. Chan, MBBS (Hons) FRANZCO
Vision Eye Institute, School of Optometry and Vision Science, University of New South Wales,
270 Victoria Ave, Chatswood, Sydney,
NSW 2067, Australia
e-mail: colin.chan@visioneyeinstitute.com.au

C. Chan (ed.), *Dry Eye: A Practical Approach*, Essentials in Ophthalmology,
DOI 10.1007/978-3-662-44106-0_3, © Springer-Verlag Berlin Heidelberg 2015

Table 3.1 Specialized and nonspecialized tests for MGD and MGD-related disease

Testing category	Specific test(s)	Tests for a general clinic	Tests for a specialized unit
Symptoms			
	Questionnaires	McMonnies, Schein, OSDI, DEQ, OCI, SPEED, and others	McMonnies, Schein, OSDI, DEQ, OCI, SPEED, and others
Signs			
Meibomian function	Lid morphology	Slit lamp microscopy	Slit lamp microscopy, confocal microscopy
	Meibomian gland mass	Slit lamp microscopy	Meibography
	Gland expressibility, expressed oil quality and volume	Interferometry, slit lamp	Slit lamp microscopy
	Lid margin reservoir		
	Tear film lipid layer, thickness, spread time, spread rate		
Evaporation tears	Evaporimetry		Evaporimetry
Osmolarity	Osmolarity	TearLab device, others	TearLab device, others
Stability	Tear film	TFBUT, ocular protection index	TFBUT, ocular protection index
	Tear film lipid layer	Spread time	Interferometry, spread rate, pattern
Indices of volume and secretion	Tear secretion	Schirmer 1	Fluorophotometry/fluorescein clearance rate
	Tear volume	Not available	Volume by fluorophotometry
	Tear volume	Meniscus height	Meniscus radius of curvature, meniscometry
	Tear clearance	Tear film index	Tear film index
Ocular surface	Ocular surface staining	Oxford scheme; NEI/industry scheme	Oxford scheme, NEI/industry scheme
Inflammation	Biomarkers		Flow cytometry, bead arrays, microarrays, mass spectrometry, cytokines and other mediators, interleukins, matrix metalloproteinases

Reprinted with permission from Nichols et al. (2011)

Tests of glandular function are presented first followed by those related disorders such as dry eye

OSDI ocular surface disease index, *DEQ* dry eye questionnaire, *OCI* ocular comfort index, *SPEED* standard patient evaluation of eye dryness

Key Questions Are

1. What are key symptoms of dry eye experienced?
2. What is the severity of the dry eye?
3. Is this evaporative tear loss (meibomian gland dysfunction) or is this aqueous deficiency (Sjogren's syndrome)?
4. Is there any underlying cause that needs additional treatment and investigation?

3.2 Answering the Key Questions

3.2.1 Key Question 1: Identify and Rank Key Symptoms

- Use a validated dry eye questionnaire such as the OSDI (Ocular Surface Disease Index Table 3.3) (Schiffman et al. 2000).
- Use your own personal standard modified questionnaire with severity scores so that an

Table 3.2 Current diagnostic methods

Recommended diagnostic tests	Identify symptoms	Determine severity	Differentiate between evaporative & aqueous
Questionnaire	X	X	X
Schirmers 1		X	X
Tear film break up time		X	X
Corneal staining		X	X
Lid margin exam		X	X

objective rating can be generated. For an example, see Table 3.4.

- This can be easily filled out by the patient in the waiting room and saves your time during the consultation.
- Allows you to monitor objectively the success of treatment.

3.2.2 Key Question 2: Determine the Severity of Dry Eye

- The questionnaire (as above) will allow you to gauge severity based on symptoms.
- The three signs recommended and traditionally used are:
  A. Schirmer 1, i.e., Schirmer without anesthetic
  B. Tear film break-up time (TFBUT) with fluorescein
  C. Corneal staining with fluorescein

3.2.2.1 Tips
A. Schirmer 1.
  - Schirmer 1 tends to be more useful if positive, i.e., less than 10 mm of strip wetting. Scores of above 10 show less repeatability. Therefore, a Schirmer appears to be more useful in advanced disease (Nichols et al. 2004).

- I typically do the Schirmer 1 test at the initial consultation to determine the severity of the dry eye and whether aqueous dysfunction exists but find it an unreliable method for monitoring treatment success. TFBUT seems to be a better method of monitoring treatment success.
- *Performance of Schirmer test* (Kaštelan et al. 2013; DEWS 2007):
  - Place the Schirmer strip between the junction of the middle and outer third of the lower lid (Fig. 3.1).
  - Ask the patient to close their eyes.
  - Note the time.
  - Remove the strips after 5 min, or until the strips are completely saturated with tears, if sooner.
B. TFBUT.
  - TFBUT values can differ greatly depending on method of fluorescein instillation, i.e., type and concentration of fluorescein used and time elapsed since fluorescein instilled.
  - TFBUT was found to become sensitive and specific as an indicator of dry eye than tear osmolarity the more severe the dry eye is (Lemp et al. 2011).

Table 3.3 Image courtesy of Allergan, Inc

Ocular Surface Disease Index© (OSDI©)[2]

Ask your patients the following 12 questions, and circle the number in the box that best represents each answer. Then, fill in boxes A, B, C, D, and E according to the instructions beside each.

Have you experienced any of the following *during the last week*?	All of the time	Most of the time	Half of the time	Some of the time	None of the time
1. Eyes that are sensitive to light? . .	4	3	2	1	0
2. Eyes that feel gritty?	4	3	2	1	0
3. Painful or sore eyes?	4	3	2	1	0
4. Blurred vision?	4	3	2	1	0
5. Poor vision?	4	3	2	1	0

Subtotal score for answers 1 to 5 **(A)**

Have problems with your eyes limited you in performing any of the following *during the last week*?	All of the time	Most of the time	Half of the time	Some of the time	None of the time	N/A
6. Reading?	4	3	2	1	0	N/A
7. Driving at night?	4	3	2	1	0	N/A
8. Working with a computer or bank machine (ATM)?	4	3	2	1	0	N/A
9. Watching TV?	4	3	2	1	0	N/A

Subtotal score for answers 6 to 9 **(B)**

Have your eyes felt uncomfortable in any of the following situations *during the last week*?	All of the time	Most of the time	Half of the time	Some of the time	None of the time	N/A
10. Windy conditions?	4	3	2	1	0	N/A
11. Places or areas with low humidity (very dry)?	4	3	2	1	0	N/A
12. Areas that are air conditioned? . . .	4	3	2	1	0	N/A

Subtotal score for answers 10 to 12 **(C)**

Add subtotals A, B, and C to obtain D
(D = sum of scores for all questions answered) **(D)**

Total number of questions answered
(do not include questions answered N/A) **(E)**

Please turn over the questionnaire to calculate the patient's final OSDI© score.

Table 3.3 (continued)

Evaluating the OSDI© Score[1]

The OSDI© is assessed on a scale of 0 to 100, with higher scores representing greater disability. The index demonstrates sensitivity and specificity in distinguishing between normal subjects and patients with dry eye disease. The OSDI© is a valid and reliable instrument for measuring dry eye disease (normal, mild to moderate, and severe) and effect on vision-related function.

Assessing Your Patient's Dry Eye Disease[1, 2]

Use your answers D and E from side 1 to compare the sum of scores for all questions answered (D) and the number of questions answered (E) with the chart below.* Find where your patient's score would fall. Match the corresponding shade of red to the key below to determine whether your patient's score indicates normal, mild, moderate, or severe dry eye disease.

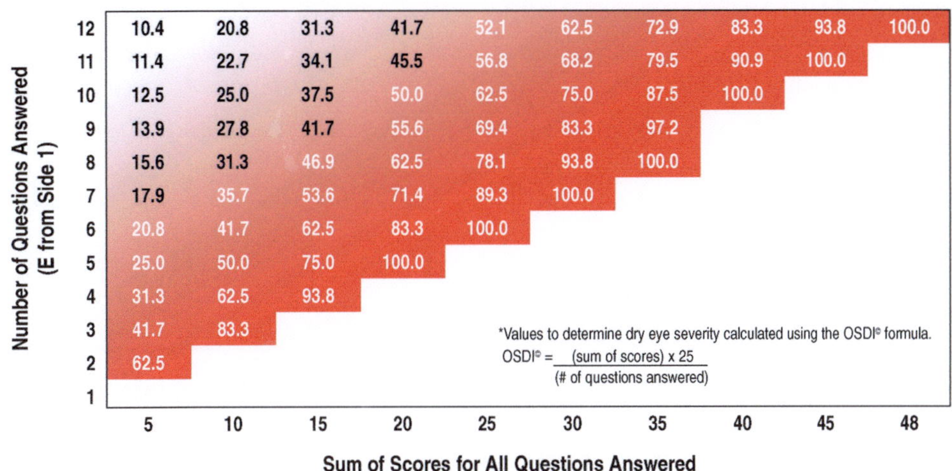

Patient's Name: ____ Date: _______________________________

How long has the patient experienced dry eye disease? ____

Eye Care Professional's Comments: ____

____

____

____

____

1. Data on file, Allergan, Inc.
2. Schiffman RM, Christianson MD, Jacobsen G, Hirsch JD, Reis BL. Reliability and validity of the Ocular Surface Disease Index. *Arch Ophthalmol.* 2000;118:615-621

Table 3.4 Dry eye questionnaire

Dr. "X" Dry eye questionnaire					
Symptom	None of the time (0)	Some of the time (1)	Most of the time (2)	All of the time (3)	Score
Do you have eyes that feel gritty/dry/burning/sensitive to light?					
Do you have fluctuating vision?					
Do your eyes feel uncomfortable if you read?					
Do your eyes feel uncomfortable if you watch TV?					
Do your eyes feel more uncomfortable in wind or air conditioning?					
				Total	

- *Performance of TFBUT* (Kaštelan et al. 2013; DEWS 2007):
- Apply one drop of 0.5 % fluorescein dye to the conjunctival fornix of each eye.
- Ask patient to blink strongly to squeeze out the excess dye.
- Wait 2 min for the fluorescein to diffuse and stain the pre-corneal tear film and tear meniscus.
- Ask the patient to blink once and hold their eyes open.
- The TFBUT is the number of seconds between the patient's last blink and the first appearance of a random dry spot on the cornea (Fig. 3.2).
- Three consecutive readings should be taken for each eye and the mean value recorded.

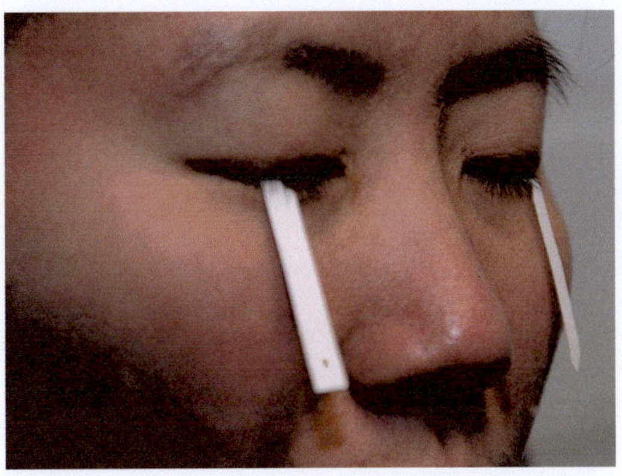

Fig. 3.1 Place the Schirmer strip between the junction of the middle and outer third of the lower lid

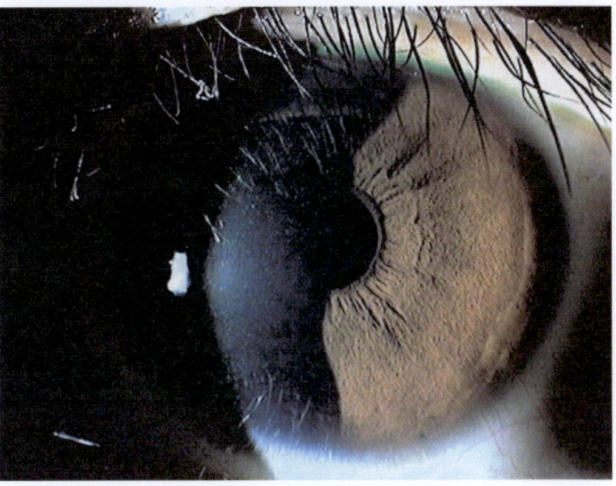

Fig. 3.3 Note and count punctate epithelial erosions/PEE

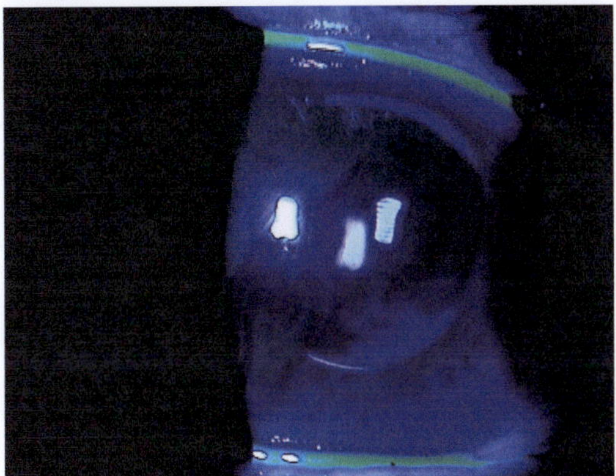

Fig. 3.2 The TFBUT is the number of seconds between the patient's last blink and the first appearance of a random dry spot on the cornea

- Add another point up to a maximum of 6:
- If PEE occur in the visual axis (central 3 mm of the cornea)
- If one or more patches of confluent staining are seen anywhere on the cornea
- If one or more corneal filaments are seen anywhere on the cornea

3.2.3 Key Question 3: Differentiate Between Meibomian Gland Dysfunction/MGD (Evaporative) and Sjogren's (Aqueous) (Tong et al. 2010)

C. Corneal staining with fluorescein.
- The presence of any corneal staining according to the DEWS classification indicates already moderate to severe dry eye. Therefore, any corneal staining should be a red flag even if the patient is minimally symptomatic.
- *Performance of corneal staining* (Kaštelan et al. 2013; DEWS 2007):
  - Perform steps outlined for TFBUT.
  - Note and count punctate epithelial erosions/PEE (Fig. 3.3).
  - If 1–5 PEE are seen, the corneal score is 1; if 6–30 PEE are seen, the score is 2; if >30 PEE are seen, the score is 3.

> **Remember MGD accounts for the vast majority of dry.**
> - Dry eye symptoms that get worse with wind/air conditioning are more indicative of an evaporative issue.
> - Which of the two signs (Schirmer versus TFBUT) is lower will indicate which is the more likely cause. In severe dry eye states, both signs will have low scores as primary aqueous deficiency will cause secondary meibomian gland dysfunction and vice versa.
> - Serology testing and questioning about associated dry mouth/joint issues may

help diagnose Sjogren's though serology has a high false-negative rate (about 20 %). It is worthwhile retesting for Sjogren's after a few years as patients can become seropositive. Consider a salivary gland biopsy if serology is negative and you or the patient want to pursue a definitive diagnosis (Qin et al. 2013).

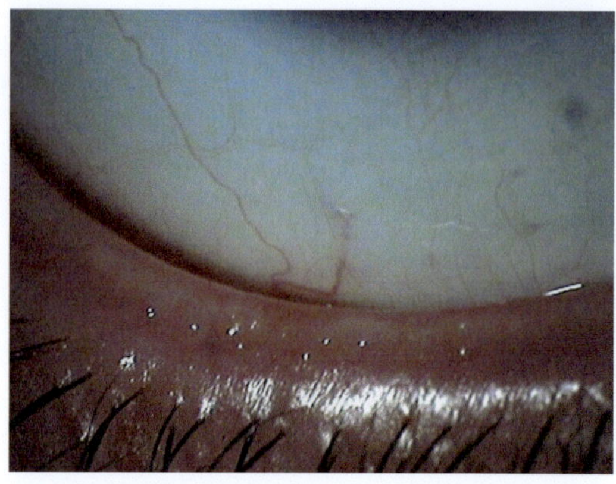

Fig. 3.4 Blocked meibomian gland orifices

D. Examination of the lid margin.

The upper and lower lid margin should be examined closely for the following signs:

- Blepharitis/scale
- Blocked meibomian gland orifices (Fig. 3.4)
- Expressibility (Table 3.5)
- Vascularization
- Lid notching (Fig. 3.5)

Vascularization and lid notching are signs of severe and chronic MGD. Vascularization may be more pronounced in ocular rosacea. Lid notching indicates meibomian gland atrophy, which is the end result of chronic MGD.

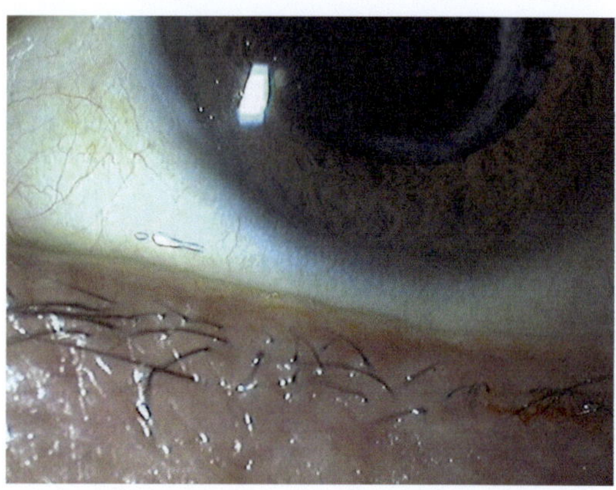

Fig. 3.5 Lid notching

Table 3.5 Clinical summary of the MGD staging used to guide treatment

Stage	MGD grade	Symptoms	Corneal staining
1	+ (minimally altered expressibility and secretion quality)	None	None
2	++ (mildly altered expressibility and secretion quality)	Minimal to mild	None to limited
3	+++ (moderately altered expressibility and secretion quality)	Moderate	Mild to moderate; mainly peripheral
4	++++ (severely altered expressibility and secretion quality)	Marked	Marked; central in addition
"Plus" disease	Coexisting or accompanying disorders of the ocular surface and/or eyelids		

Reprinted with permission from Nichols et al. (2011)

3.2.3.1 Meibomian Gland Expression or Expressibility

Meibomian gland expression or expressibility is recommended as part of the standard examination of dry eye. Korb et al. demonstrated that there is a correlation between the number of meibomian glands yielding a liquid secretion when expressed (Korb and Blackie 2008).

However, meibomian gland expression has potentially the most visit-to-visit and interobserver variability unless a device such as the Korb expressor is used to apply a standard degree of force to the eyelid over a defined area. Expression with the index finger applied to the lower lid has been described previously (see below), but clearly it is impossible to exactly replicate the same amount of pressure over the same area consistently every time (Meadows et al. 2012).

3.2.3.2 Proposed Standard Technique

1. Ideally use a device such as the Korb expressor which applies a standard degree of force (1.25 g/mm^2) over a standard area (8.76 mm $\times$ 4.45 mm $= 38.95$ mm^2).
2. If such a device is not available, then apply external firm pressure with a fingertip, rod, paddle, or spatula for 10–15 s to the central meibomian glands. It has been estimated that the pressure elicited by a standardized device is equivalent to that necessary to elevate IOP to 30 mmHg (Tomlinson et al. 2011).
3. Meibomian gland expressibility and secretions can be graded according to Table 3.5.

3.2.4 Key Question 4: Is There Any Underlying Cause That Needs Additional Treatment and Investigation?

E. Assess the conjunctiva to determine if there is an unusual underlying cause.

It is a common error in a busy clinic to neglect this part of the examination.

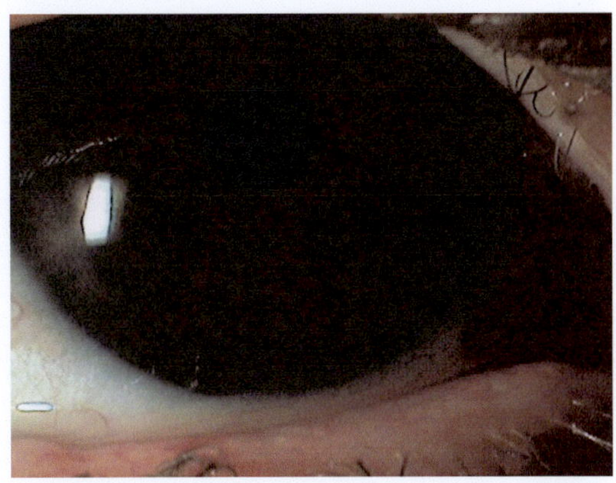

Fig. 3.6 Conjunctivochalasis

Suggested Steps in Examining the Conjunctiva
- The lower lid should be pulled down and the inferior cul de sac should be examined specifically for signs such as:
    - Symblepharon (ocular cicatricial pemphigoid and Stevens-Johnson syndrome).
    - Conjunctivochalasis (Fig. 3.6). Patient should be asked to look down as conjunctivochalasis may become more obvious in downward gaze.
- The upper lid should be pulled up while the patient is looking down to examine for signs such as
    - Dilated superior conjunctival vessels (superior limbic keratoconjunctivitis/SLK)
    - Trabeculectomy bleb
- The upper lid should be everted to examine the tarsal conjunctiva for signs such as:
    - Trachoma scarring/Arlt's line (Fig. 3.7)
    - Papillae (allergy/contact lens hypersensitivity)

F. Examine the cornea for signs of the underlying cause, masquerade syndromes, and corneal damage such as
- Marginal ulcers/scars (blepharitis/rosacea)
- Geographic subepithelial lines (anterior basement membrane dystrophy or map-dot-fingerprint dystrophy; see Fig. 3.8)

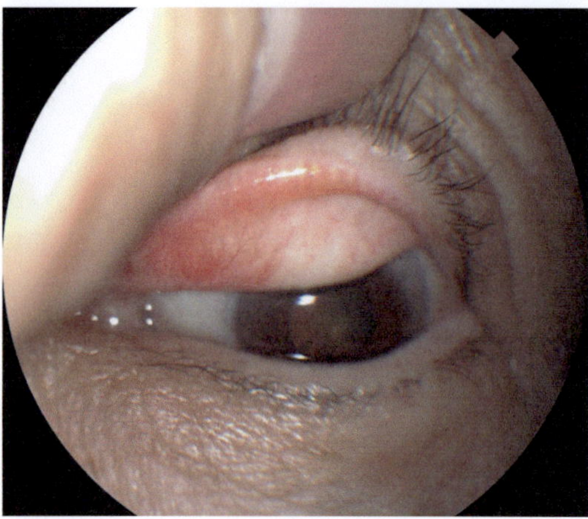

Fig. 3.7 Trachoma scarring/Arlt's line

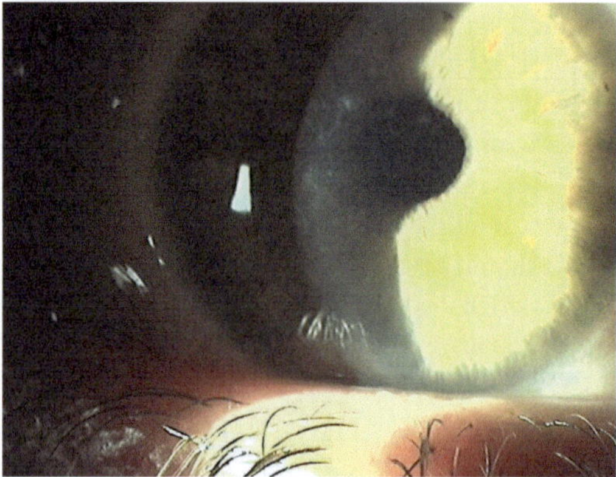

Fig. 3.8 Geographic subepithelial lines (anterior basement membrane dystrophy or map-dot-fingerprint dystrophy)

Common masquerade syndromes in my experience are:
- Allergy
- Anterior basement membrane dystrophy or map-dot-fingerprint dystrophy

G. Examine the head and neck region for signs of associated conditions.
- Thyroid eye disease such as exophthalmos or lid retraction
- Rosacea as facial telangiectasia

H. Questions about associated systemic conditions and risk factors.

While this is the last section on the topic of determining underlying causes, practically questions about possible associated systemic conditions and risk factors should be incorporated into the patient questionnaire or asked as part of the clinical history before the examination.

Table 3.6 outlines the known and postulated risk factors for dry eye.

The purpose of your diagnostic workup should be to guide management.

A standardized consistent approach will allow the clinician to more effectively and efficiently manage dry eye.

Using the results from the diagnostic testing and the Delphi approach (Table 3.7), dry eye can be graded into different levels of severity (grades 1, 2, 3, and 4). The international task force guidelines for dry eye therapy (Table 3.8) can then be applied appropriately.

> **Case Example**
> - Patient has constant symptoms with visual blurring, central corneal staining, TFBUT, and Schirmer score less than 5 = grade 3.
> - Grade 3 level therapy would include level 1 therapy measures + level 2 therapy measures then level 3 if level 2 therapies fail.
> - A typical patient would already be on artificial tears, lid margin treatment such as warm compress, and omega 3 supplements. Topical steroids and oral tetracyclines may be tried next followed by punctual occlusion.

3.3 Newer Diagnostic Technologies

There are a number of newer diagnostic techniques for dry eye. At this point at time, it is not recommended as part of standard diagnostics but these technologies are novel and may evolve. Cost may be a factor as well as to whether you

Table 3.6 Risk factors for dry eye

Level of evidence		
Mostly consistent[a]	Suggestive[b]	Unclear[c]
Older age	Asian race	Cigarette smoking
Female sex	Medications	Hispanic ethnicity
	Tricyclic antidepressants	
	Selective serotonin reuptake inhibitors	
	Diuretics	
	Beta-blockers	
Postmenopausal estrogen therapy		
Omega-3 and omega-6 fatty acids		Anticholinergics
		Anxiolytics
		Antipsychotics
		Alcohol
Medications		
Antihistimines		
Connective tissue disease	Diabetes mellitus	
LASIK and refractive excimer laser surgery	HIV/HTLV1 infection	Menopause
Radiation therapy	Systemic chemotherapy	Botulinum toxin injection
Hematopoietic stem cell transplantation	Large incision ECCE and penetrating keratoplasty	
	Isotretinoin	Acne
Vitamin A deficiency	Low humidity environments	Gout
Hepatitis C infection	Sarcoidosis	Oral contraceptives
Androgen deficiency	Ovarian dysfunction	Pregnancy

Reprinted with permission from The Epidemiology of Dry eye Disease. Report of the Epidemiology Subcommittee of the International Dry eye Workshop (2007)

[a]Mostly consistent evidence implies the existence of at least one adequately powered and otherwise well-conducted study published in a peer-reviewed journal along with the existence of a plausible biological rationale and corroborating basic research or clinical data

[b]Suggestive evidence implies the existence of either: (1) inconclusive information from peer-reviewed publications or (2) inconclusive or limited information to support the association, but either not published or published somewhere other than in a peer-reviewed journal

[c]Unclear evidence implies either directly conflicting information in peer-reviewed publications or inconclusive information but with some basis for a biological rationale

decide to incorporate them into your clinic. This section does not discuss all newer diagnostic technologies; only few which are more commonly used and have reasonable peer-reviewed evidence to support their use.

3.3.1 Tear Osmolarity

A hyperosmolar tear film is thought to be a core component of the pathophysiology of dry eye. A relatively new device, the Tearlab, is a commercial instrument that measures the osmolarity of tears collected via capillary action along a thin strip. This strip is then inserted into a measuring device (Fig. 3.9).

A prospective multicenter trial showed that tear osmolarity showed sensitivity and specificity comparable if not better than traditional tests for detecting dry eye in mild to moderate cases. However, TFBUT was a better indicator for more severe cases of dry eye. A major issue with the TearLab is that it shows relatively poor repeatability (Lemp et al. 2011; Kaštelan et al. 2013; Garcia et al. 2014).

Table 3.7 Dry eye severity grading scheme

Dry eye severity level	1	2	3	4[a]
Discomfort, severity, and frequency	Mild and/or episodic occurs under environ stress	Moderate episodic or chronic, stress or no stress	Severe frequent or constant without stress	Severe and/or disabling and constant
Visual symptoms	None or episodic mild fatigue	Annoying and/or activity limiting episodic	Annoying, chronic, and/or constant limiting activity	Constant and/or possibly disabling
Conjunctival injection	None to mild	None to mild	+/−	+/++
Conjunctival staining	None to mild	Variable	Moderate to marked	Marked
Corneal staining (severity/location)	None to mild	Variable	Marked central	Severe punctate erosions
Corneal/tear signs	None to mild	Mild debris, ↓ meniscus	Filamentary keratitis, mucus clumping, ↑ tear debris	Filamentary keratitis, mucus clumping, ↑ tear debris, ulceration
Lid/meibomian glands	MGD variably present	MGD variably present	Frequent	Trichiasis, keratinization, symblepharon
TFBUT (s)	Variable	≤10	≤5	Immediate
Schirmer score (mm/5 min)	Variable	≤10	≤5	≤2

Reprinted with permission from Management and Therapy of Dry Eye Disease: Report of the Management and Therapy Subcommittee of the International Dry Eye Workshop (2007)
TBUT fluorescein tear break-up time, *MGD* meibomian gland disease
[a]Must have signs and symptoms

Table 3.8 Treatment recommendations for DTS on the basis of level of severity

DTS severity	Treatment recommendations	
Level 1	No treatment	Use of hypoallergenic products
	Preserved tears	Water intake
	Environmental management	Psychological support
	Allergy drops	Avoidance of drugs contributing to dry eye
Level 2	Unpreserved tears	Secretagogues
	Gels	Topical steroids
	Ointments	Topical cyclosporine A
	Nutritional support (flaxseed/fatty acids)	
Level 3	Tetracyclines	
	Punctal plugs	
Level 4	Surgery	Punctal cautery
	Systemic anti-inflammatory therapy	Acetylcysteine
	Oral cyclosporine	Contact lenses
	Moisture goggles	

Reprinted with permission from Management and Therapy of Dry Eye Disease: Report of the Management and Therapy Subcommittee of the International Dry Eye Workshop (2007)

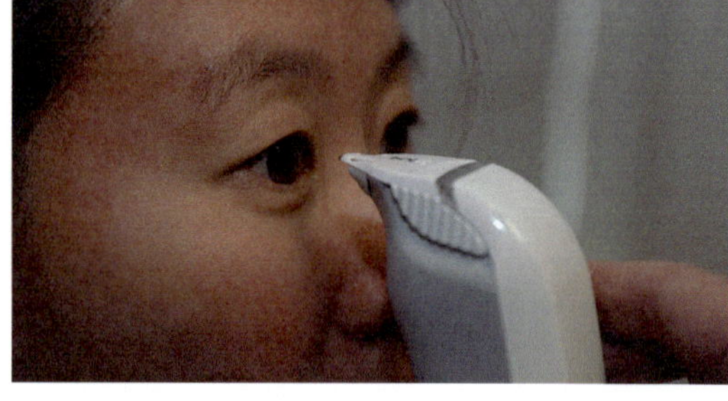

Fig. 3.9 The TearLab is a commercial instrument that measures the osmolarity of tears collected via capillary action along a thin strip. This strip is then inserted into a measuring device

3.3.2 Interferometry

Tear film interferometry is not a new diagnostic test. Interferometry involves the use of infrared light interference patterns to produce a qualitative image of the tear lipid layer (Fig. 3.10). However, newer devices are able to measure the actual thickness of the lipid layer as well as have built-in software to give a computerized TFBUT measure. These devices can be an excellent educational tool for patients but have

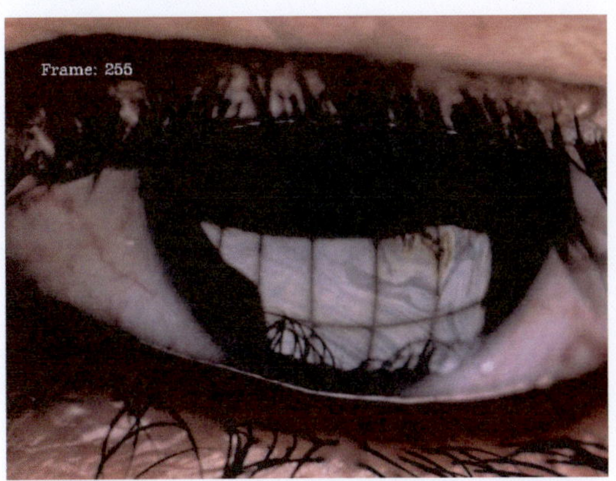

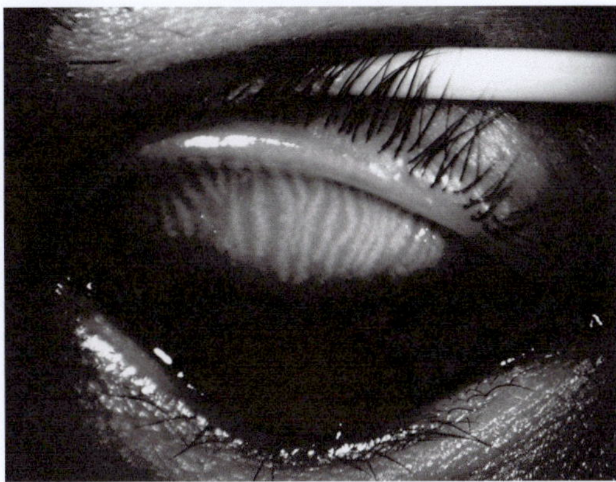

Fig. 3.10 Interferometry involves the use of infrared light interference patterns to produce a qualitative image of the tear lipid layer

Fig. 3.11 Imaging of the meibomian glands through transillumination or infrared devices to date has mainly been performed in university research labs

not yet supplanted the simpler TFBUT with fluorescein (Eom et al. 2013; Hosaka et al. 2011).

3.3.3 Meibography

Imaging of the meibomian glands through transillumination or infrared devices to date has mainly been performed in university research labs (Fig. 3.11). However, some commercial devices are emerging. Imaging can be useful in determining how likely treatment is going to work. For example, the atrophied meibomian glands are unlikely to respond to any treatment modality. It does not require meibography to tell you a gland has atrophied, as lid notching is a good clinical indication that this has happened (*Arita 2013; Ban et al. 2013; Pult and Riede-Pult 2013).

3.4 Summary

In summary, it is crucial to have a standardized approach to the diagnosis of dry eye. Standard testing should include a questionnaire, tear film break-up time (TBUT), Schirmer test, and corneal staining with fluorescein. It is also important to look for and consider coexistent conditions, both ocular and systemic, which may be causing or exacerbating the dry eye condition.

Standardized testing then allows standardized grading and standardized management with the Delphi approach. With such an approach, successful treatment is more likely to occur.

Compliance with Ethical Requirements

Colin Chan declares that he has no conflict of interest.

All procedures followed were in accordance with the ethical standards of the responsible committee on human experimentation (institutional and national) and with the Helsinki Declaration of 1975, as revised in 2000 (5). Informed consent was obtained from all patients for being included in the study.

No animal studies were carried out by the authors for this article.

References

Arita R (2013) Validity of noninvasive meibography systems: noncontact meibography equipped with a slit-lamp and a mobile pen-shaped meibograph. Cornea 32(Suppl 1):S65–S70. doi:10.1097/ICO.0b013e3182a2c7c6

Ban Y, Shimazaki-Den S, Tsubota K, Shimazaki J (2013) Morphological evaluation of meibomian glands using noncontact infrared meibography. Ocul Surf 11(1):47–53. doi:10.1016/j.jtos.2012.09.005, Epub 2012 Oct 16

Diagnostic Methodology Subcommittee of the International Dry Eye WorkShop (DEWS) (2007) Methodologies to diagnose and monitor dry eye disease: report of the Diagnostic Methodology Subcommittee of the International Dry Eye WorkShop (2007). Ocul Surf 5(2):108–152

Downie LE, Keller PR, Vingrys AJ (2013) An evidence-based analysis of Australian optometrists' dry eye practices. Optom Vis Sci 90(12):1385–1395. doi:10.1097/OPX.0000000000000087

Eom Y, Lee JS, Kang SY, Kim HM, Song JS (2013) Correlation between quantitative measurements of tear film lipid layer thickness and meibomian gland loss in patients with obstructive meibomian gland dysfunction and normal controls. Am J Ophthalmol 155(6):1104–1110.e2. doi:10.1016/j.ajo.2013.01.008, Epub 2013 Mar 7

García N, Tesón M, Enríquez-de-Salamanca A, Mena L, Sacristán A, Fernández I, Calonge M, González-García MJ (2014) Basal values, intra-day and inter-day variations in tear film osmolarity and tear fluorescein clearance. Curr Eye Res 8

Gayton J (2009) Etiology, prevalence, and treatment of dry eye disease. Clin Ophthalmol 3:405–412

Hosaka E, Kawamorita T, Ogasawara Y, Nakayama N, Uozato H, Shimizu K, Dogru M, Tsubota K, Goto E (2011) Interferometry in the evaluation of precorneal tear film thickness in dry eye. Am J Ophthalmol 151(1):18–23.e1. doi:10.1016/j.ajo.2010.07.019

Kaštelan S, Tomic M, Salopek-Rabatic J, Novak B (2013) Diagnostic procedures and management of dry eye. Biomed Res Int 2013:309723. doi:10.1155/2013/309723, Epub 2013 Aug 19

Korb DR, Blackie CA (2008) Meibomian gland diagnostic expressibility: correlation with dry eye symptoms and gland location. Cornea 27(10):1142–1147. doi:10.1097/ICO.0b013e3181814cff

Lemp MA, Bron AJ, Baudouin C, Benítez Del Castillo JM, Geffen D, Tauber J, Foulks GN, Pepose JS, Sullivan BD (2011) Tear osmolarity in the diagnosis and management of dry eye disease. Am J Ophthalmol 151(5):792–798.e1. doi:10.1016/j.ajo.2010.10.032, Epub 2011 Feb 18

Levinson BA, Rapuano CJ, Cohen EJ, Hammersmith KM, Ayres BD, Laibson PR (2008) Referrals to the Wills Eye Institute Cornea Service after laser in situ keratomileusis: reasons for patient dissatisfaction. J Cataract Refract Surg 34(1):32–39. doi:10.1016/j.jcrs.2007.08.028

Management and therapy of dry eye disease: report of the Management and Therapy Subcommittee of the International Dry Eye Workshop (2007) Ocul Surf 5(2):163–178

Meadows JF, Ramamoorthy P, Nichols JJ, Nichols KK (2012) Development of the 4-3-2-1 meibum expressibility scale. Eye Contact Lens 38(2):86–92. doi:10.1097/ICL.0b013e318242b494

Nettune GR, Pflugfelder SC (2010) Post-LASIK tear dysfunction and dysesthesia. Ocul Surf 8(3):135–145, Review

Nichols KK, Mitchell GL, Zadnik K (2004) The repeatability of clinical measurements of dry eye. Cornea 23(3):272–285

Nichols KK, Foulks GN, Bron AJ, Glasgow BJ, Dogru M, Tsubota K, Lemp MA, Sullivan DA (2011) The international workshop on meibomian gland dysfunction: executive summary. Invest Ophthalmol Vis Sci 52(4):1922–1929. doi:10.1167/iovs.10-6997a

Pult H, Riede-Pult B (2013) Comparison of subjective grading and objective assessment in meibography. Cont Lens Anterior Eye 36(1):22–27. doi:10.1016/j.clae.2012.10.074, Epub 2012 Oct 27

Qin Q, Wang H, Wang HZ, Huang YL, Li H, Zhang WW, Zhang JR, He LL, Xia R, Zhao DB, Deng AM (2014) Diagnostic accuracy of anti-alpha-fodrin antibodies for primary Sjogren's syndrome. Mod Rheumatol 24(5):793–797

Reddy P, Grad O, Rajagopalan K (2004) The economic burden of dry eye: a conceptual framework and preliminary assessment. Cornea 23(8):751–761

Schiffman RM, Christianson MD, Jacobsen G, Hirsch JD, Reis BL (2000) Reliability and validity of the Ocular Surface Disease Index. Arch Ophthalmol 118(5):615–621

Solomon KD, Fernández de Castro LE, Sandoval HP, Biber JM, Groat B, Neff KD, Ying MS, French JW, Donnenfeld ED, Lindstrom RL, Joint LASIK Study Task Force (2009) LASIK world literature review: quality of life and patient satisfaction. Ophthalmology 116(4):691–701. doi:10.1016/j.ophtha.2008.12.037, Review

The Epidemiology of Dry Eye Disease. Report of the Epidemiology Subcommittee of the International Dry eye Workshop (2007) (2007) Ocul Surf 5(2):93–107

Tomlinson A, Bron AJ, Korb DR, Amano S, Paugh JR, Pearce EI, Yee R, Yokoi N, Arita R, Dogru M (2011) The International Workshop on Meibomian Gland Dysfunction: report of the Diagnosis Subcommittee. Invest Ophthalmol Vis Sci 52:2006–2049. doi:10.1167/iovs.10-6997f

Tong L, Waduthantri S, Wong TY, Saw SM, Wang JJ, Rosman M, Lamoreux E (2010) Impact of symptomatic dry eye on vision-related daily activities: the Singapore Malay Eye Study. Eye (Lond) 24(9):1486–1491. doi:10.1038/eye.2010.67, Epub 2010 May 21

Woodward MA, Randleman JB, Stulting RD (2009) Dissatisfaction after multifocal intraocular lens implantation. J Cataract Refract Surg 35(6):992–997. doi:10.1016/j.jcrs.2009.01.031

Yu J, Asche CV, Fairchild CJ (2011) The economic burden of dry eye disease in the United States: a decision tree analysis. Cornea 30(4):379–387. doi:10.1097/ICO.0b013e3181f7f363

Artificial Tears

4

Renato Ambrósio Jr, Fernando Faria Correia, Isaac Ramos, and Marcella Salomão

The mainstay treatment of dry eye or dysfunctional tear syndrome (DTS) is tear replacement with artificial tears (AT). However, the term "artificial tears" may be considered as a misnomer, as the products available still do not mimic the composition of human tears and function as ocular surface lubricants. In fact the purpose of ATs is to reduce clinical signs and symptoms and to protect the ocular surface (Schaumberg et al. 2003). The ability of each drug to accomplish these purposes depends on physical properties associated to its formulation and on its mechanism of action. There are different products available as AT, whose ability to accomplish ocular surface lubrication depends on the physical properties and mechanism of action associated to the composition of each formulation.

ATs are typically hypotonic or isotonic buffered solutions that are usually commercialized as over-the-counter (OTC) products. Tear substitute formulations are usually commonly found as preserved, multidose preparations. However, preservative-free systems are available as unit-dose vials (Fig. 4.1) or as multidose containers such as the ABAK® and COMOD® (Fig. 4.2) systems.

AT consists of an active ingredient that promotes ocular surface wetting, buffering agents, preservatives, electrolytes, and other factors that vary widely from product to product. There are a variety of AT products on the market with different characteristics that may differently benefit specific types of ocular surface and tear dysfunction cases. The concept of customization of AT is related to an advanced understanding of the ocular surface and tear film and to the properties of different compounds available on AT. Specific deficiencies may be detected on each patient, to that an optimized AT selection is possible for enhancing patient benefit.

R. Ambrósio Jr, MD, PhD (✉)
Cornea and Refractive Surgery, Instituto de Olhos
Renato Ambrósio, Room 702, 211 Conde do Bonfim
Street, Rio de Janeiro, RJ 20520-050, Brazil

Rio de Janeiro Corneal Tomography and
Biomechanics Study Group, Rio de Janeiro, Brazil

Department of Ophthalmology, Federal University
of Sao Paulo, Sao Paulo, Brazil
e-mail: dr.renatoambrosio@gmail.com

F.F. Correia, MD
Rio de Janeiro Corneal Tomography and
Biomechanics Study Group, Rio de Janeiro, Brazil

Department of Ophthalmology, University of Porto,
Porto, Portugal
e-mail: f.faria.correia@gmail.com

I. Ramos, MD
Rio de Janeiro Corneal Tomography and
Biomechanics Study Group, Rio de Janeiro, Brazil

Cataract and Refractive Surgery, Hospital de Olhos
Santa Luzia, Gruta de Lourdes,
Maceió, Alagoas, Brazil
e-mail: isaacramos_@hotmail.com

M. Salomão, MD
Rio de Janeiro Corneal Tomography and
Biomechanics Study Group, Rio de Janeiro, Brazil

Department of Ophthalmology, Federal University
of Sao Paulo, Sao Paulo, Brazil
e-mail: marcella@nhtelecom.com.br

C. Chan (ed.), *Dry Eye: A Practical Approach*, Essentials in Ophthalmology,
DOI 10.1007/978-3-662-44106-0_4, © Springer-Verlag Berlin Heidelberg 2015

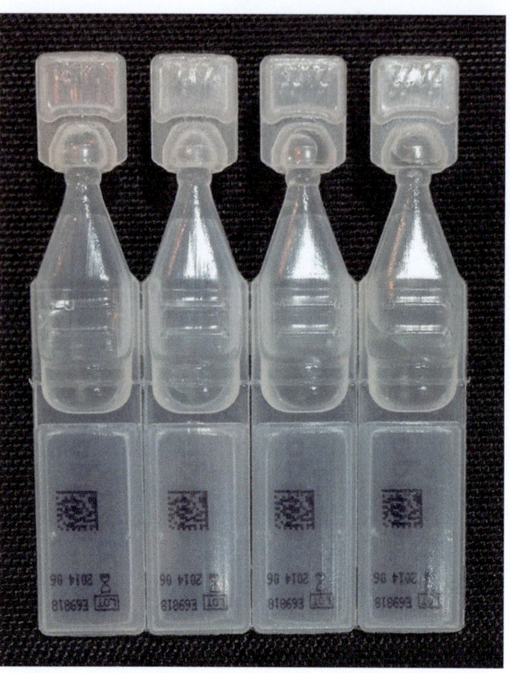

Fig. 4.1 Preservative-free unit-dose vials

Components of ATs
- Active ingredient to promote ocular surface wetting
- Buffering agents
- Preservatives
- Electrolytes

Properties
- Reduce clinical signs and symptoms.
- Protect ocular surface.
- Promote ocular surface wetting.

Various diagnostic measures are used to specify the best indication and to determine the efficacy of an AT. Tear film breakup time (TFBUT), corneal and conjunctival vital dye staining, and symptom questionnaires are among the most common measures. Objective information from systems as the

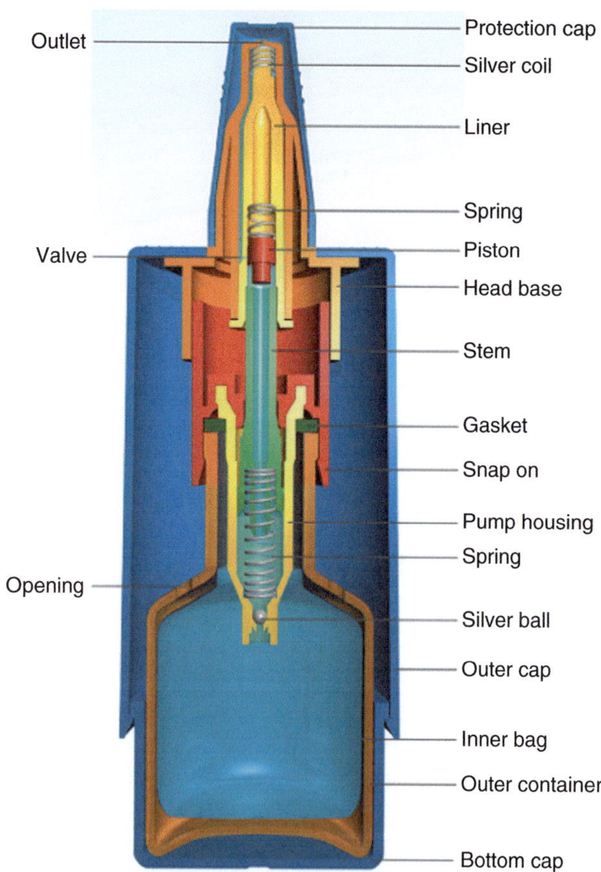

Fig. 4.2 COMOD® system for preservative-free multidose containers

Keratograph 5 (Oculus, Wetzlar, Germany) helps to evaluate tear substitute treatments. This chapter reviews the basics for understanding the most common formulations available for AT.

> - Most dry eye sufferers primarily manage their dry eye with OTC artificial tears (AT) or tear substitute eyedrops
> - It is estimated that over ten million Americans use AT.
> - Different ATs are available on the market with different properties.

4.1 General Aspects of Tear Substitutes

4.1.1 Viscosity Properties

Viscosity, or fluid thickness, has been considered one of the most important properties of an AT. Higher viscosity leads to longer retention of the agent in the ocular surface, which is beneficial in terms of relieving the signs and symptoms related to dry eye or dysfunctional tear syndrome. However, the thicker constitution is prone to cause blurring of vision after instillation and may leave runoff residues on the eyelashes or lids as the solution dries out. The challenge for AT preparations is to accomplish a certain level of viscosity that maximizes its retention time and maintains visual clearness, thereby augmenting clinical efficacy (Bhojwani et al. 2011).

> **Increase AT Viscosity →**
> - ↑ retention time
> - ↑ residues
> - ↓ clarity of vision

4.1.2 Demulcent Agents

Demulcents are lubricating compounds contained in AT that have a mucilaginous consistency, which

Table 4.1 Categories of ophthalmic demulcents

Cellulose derivatives
Liquid polyols
Polyvinyl alcohol
Gelatin
Dextran 70
Povidone

provides lubricity for protecting and smoothing the ocular surface, thereby minimizing abrasive actions of the eyelids. The US Food and Drug Administration (FDA) recognizes six categories of ophthalmic demulcents (Table 4.1).

To be allowed in "over-the-counter" (OTC) preparations, the demulcents should fall within certain concentration ranges according to international standards. An AT may contain up to three demulcents in its preparations. An ophthalmic vasoconstrictor or a vasoconstrictor with astringent combination could be included to provide the AT with additional redness- or discomfort-reducing properties.

Cellulose derivatives are the most common demulcents found in modern tear substitutes. Their concentration range goes from 0.2 to 2.5 %. The two main cellulose derivatives available for AT preparations are hydroxypropylmethylcellulose (HPMC) and carboxymethylcellulose (CMC). Cellulose derivatives also function as viscosity agents if its concentration is increased, which prolongs its retention time in the ocular surface. Similarly, CMC preparations, typically presented in 0.5 or 1.0 % CMC, have different viscosity, with the higher concentration forming a thicker, gel-like liquid. In addition, cellulose-based demulcents can be combined with an oil in order to enhance its mucoadhesive properties, which improves either the mucin and lipid components of the tear film (Rieger 1990). CMC can also be combined with osmoprotectants such as glycerin, L-carnitine, and erythritol, which are biocompatible solutes that aim to protect cells from the physiological stress of exposure to hyperosmotic conditions. Altering these characteristics may be a strategy for deciding the concentration and composition of cellulose-derived AT in accordance with the type and severity of TDS. It has also been demonstrated in a recent study that CMC can have biological effects as it appears to stimulate the closure of epithelial cell wounds in vitro as well as re-epithelization in rabbit corneas in vivo (Garrett et al. 2008).

> - Cellulose derivatives may work as viscosity agents by increasing their concentration.
> - Cellulose demulcents could also be combined with an oil in order to enhance the mucoadhesive properties of the preparation.

Liquid polyols (polyhydric alcohols) are allowable in concentrations of 0.2–1.0 %. Polyols do not have viscosity properties and are only used as lubricants. Interestingly, a comparative study demonstrated that AT containing propylene glycol 0.3 % (PG) and polyethylene glycol 0.4 % (PEG 400) provided better lubricity and longer visual acuity maintenance than a tear containing cellulose-based demulcents. Polyols can be combined with mineral oil and phospholipids to create a stable emulsion and promote stabilization of the lipid layer, especially in patients with meibomian gland dysfunction. These patients can also benefit from lipid only containing artificial tears, such as castor oil and mineral oil.

Glycerin and polysorbate are liquid polyols that are used in different concentrations as combinative agents in oil emulsion systems for improving the lipid layer of the tear film. In addition, hydroxypropyl (HP)-guar is a gelling agent with high molecular weight derived from guar gum that is used in an AT with the demulcents PG and PEG 400. The gelling action is triggered by contact with the ocular surface, being influenced by the pH. One of the most important properties of HP-guar is its ability to hydrate very fast when in contact with cold water and to obtain high viscosity and uniformity with relative low concentrations. When in contact with the human tear film, it bonds epithelial cells, reproducing the glycocalyx structure, and this connection results

in longer maintenance of the demulcents in the ocular surface.

Polyvinyl alcohol (PVA) was one of the former demulcents incorporated in AT. They are included in AT preparations in concentrations from 0.1 to 4.0 %. PVA has been widely used isolated or in combination with another demulcent such as povidone. Gelatin is allowed in 0.01 % concentration, but not commonly used in commercial AT. Dextran 70 can only be used in AT preparations in conjunction with another demulcent agent. Dextran 70, gelatin, and povidone also have viscosity properties in addition to lubrication. Hyaluronic acid is also a viscosity agent that was initially been developed as an intraocular viscoelastic. It has been investigated as an active compound for tear substitutes for the treatment of dry eye. The theoretical mode of action is that it holds moisture and weakly adheres to epithelial surface, so that it would be retained on the ocular surface. It is also believed to have an anti-inflammatory activity. Hyaluronic acid 0.2 % has been shown to have significantly longer ocular surface residence times than 0.3 % HPMC or 1.4 % polyvinyl alcohol, for example.

4.1.3 Preservatives

Preservatives are added to artificial lubricants in order to prevent microbial growth. They can be classified as detergent, oxidative, and, more recently, ionic-buffering preservatives. Detergents have the longest running history in ophthalmology and cause bacterial death through interruption of the lipid component of cell membranes. Examples include: benzalkonium chloride (BAK), cetrimonium chloride, chlorobutanol, and polyquaternium-1 (Polyquad®). Benzalkonium chloride (BAK) is the most frequently used preservative in ophthalmic formulations. However, these antimicrobial properties are habitually accompanied by mild toxicity to the ocular surface.

Oxidative preservatives alter DNA, lipid, and protein components of bacterial cells. Reduced toxicity can be found with these preservatives when compared to detergents, especially because they are presented in low concentrations in ophthalmic preparations. Sodium perborate and stabilized oxychloro complex (SOC or Purite ®) are examples of oxidizing preservatives. The first one is neutralized by tear proteins and the second by UV exposure. Ionic-buffered preservatives represent the more recently introduced class of ophthalmic preservatives. They act in a similar way to oxidizing drugs, and it has been shown to have both antibacterial and antifungal qualities. SofZia® is the most recent preservative of this group and is a combination of boric acid, zinc, sorbitol, and propylene glycol.

> It's critical to remember that dry eye patients often already have damaged ocular surfaces, and thus, using a preserved artificial tear many times daily can be harmful. This way, the typical ocular surface inflammation present in dry eye can be aggravated by preserved tear substitutes (Shigeyasu et al. 2013).

One of the most significant advances in the treatment of dry eye was the introduction of preservative-free preparations, which allowed patients to instill lubricants more often with less concerns about toxicity.

> Patients with severe dry eye and ocular surface disease, as well as patients on multiple preserved topical medications, such as glaucoma patients, should absolutely use preservative-free formulations.

The drawbacks to the use of nonpreserved single unit-dose tear substitutes are the cost and the inconvenience of carrying several vials. Therefore, reclosable vials were introduced in the market. Less toxic preservatives such as polyquad and sodium chlorite were also introduced trying to diminish toxic effects.

4.1.4 Electrolyte Composition

Electrolytes are naturally present in physiological human fluids such as the tear film. Solutions containing electrolytes or ions have been shown to restore damaged corneal surfaces. Potassium and bicarbonate seem to be the most important ions found in most artificial tears containing electrolytes. In a rabbit model study, treatment with an electrolyte solution increased conjunctival goblet cell density, and reduced tear osmolarity as well as rose bengal staining (Gilbard and Rossi 1992).

> Bicarbonate can help in the recovery of damaged corneal epithelium and in the maintenance of ocular surface health by maintaining the mucin layer integrity. Potassium is important due to its ability to maintain corneal thickness.

4.1.5 Osmolarity/Osmolality

Dry eye patients frequently have a higher tear film osmolarity (crystalloid osmolarity) than normal patients, most likely due to evaporation in patients with lipid layer deficiency.

> Hyperosmolarity is proinflammatory and may be toxic to the ocular surface and conjunctiva, increasing damage. Therefore hypo-osmotic formulations may help.

For this reason, hypo-osmotic formulations were developed, aiming to lower the osmolarity of the tear film. Crystalloid osmolarity is related to the presence of ions, but colloidal osmolality is related to the macromolecule content and is involved in the control of water transport in tissues. Differences in osmolality interfere with the net water flow across membranes. Damaged epithelial cells usually swell in dry eye surfaces, and thus, a fluid with high colloidal osmolality can cause cell deturgescence and return to its normal structure.

4.1.6 Alkalinity

Some research studies suggest a mean pH in healthy eyes between 7.5 and 7.6. Dry eye patients tend to have higher than average tear film pH values. The protective mechanisms to reverse the increasing alkalinity in tears are the blinking and the tear production, in order to decrease pH levels. It is also presumed that artificial tear instillation has a similar protective effect.

4.2 Combined Treatment Regimens for Dry Eye

Tear substitutes are becoming gradually more efficacious at individually managing dry eye syndrome. It is critical to know the composition and properties of each artificial tear so as to enhance the efficiency of our therapy.

Among new treatment options, several pharmacological agents have been developed to stimulate secretion of lipid, mucin, or aqueous tears. Diquafosol is a uridine triphosphate-related compound that has been reported to be a P2Y2 receptor agonist, a receptor known to contribute to water transfer and mucin secretion. In rabbit studies diquafosol has been reported to promote secretion of aqueous tears from conjunctival epithelial cells and mucins from conjunctival goblet cells on the ocular surface (Matsumoto et al. 2012).

To improve signs and symptoms derived from the dry eye disease, artificial tears can also be combined with other treatment modalities, such as topical cyclosporine A, secretagogues, corticosteroids, omega-3 fatty acids supplementation, punctal plugs, autologous serum, or even surgical procedures (International Dry Eye Workshop 2007).

4.3 Summary

Artificial tears and lubricants are the mainstay in the treatment of dry eye. Demulcents and viscosity agents contained in tear substitutes lubricate and can work to fortify the mucin layer or even the lipid layer, which prevents tear film evaporation. Viscosity agents make an artificial tear thicker, allowing a longer period in the tear film and an extended interval of patient comfort. Modern artificial tears still contain antimicrobial preservatives, which can be particularly detrimental in dry eye patients. Concerning the composition of an artificial tear, other features to consider are electrolytes (these can make for a healthier tear film), osmolarity/osmolality (a tear should be slightly hypo-osmotic), and pH. In order to optimize the treatment regimen, we might need to combine other types of therapeutic modalities such as punctal plugs, topical cyclosporine, oral antibiotics, or autologous serum.

Compliance with Ethical Requirements

Conflict of Interest Authors Fernando Faria Correia, Isaac Ramos, Marcella Salomão, and Renato Ambrósio Jr declare that they have no conflict of interest.

Animals and Humans "No animal or human studies were carried out by the authors for this article."

References

Bhojwani R, Cellesi F, Maino A, Jalil A, Haider D, Noble B (2011) Treatment of dry eye: an analysis of the British Sjögren's syndrome Association comparing substitute tear viscosity and subjective efficacy. Cont Lens Anterior Eye 34:269–273

Garrett Q, Xu S, Simmons PA, Vehige J, Xie RZ, Kumar A, Flanagan JL, Zhao Z, Willcox MD (2008) Carboxymethyl cellulose stimulates rabbit corneal epithelial wound healing. Curr Eye Res 33(7):567–573

Gilbard JP, Rossi SR (1992) An electrolyte-based solution that increases corneal glycogen and conjunctival goblet-cell density in a rabbit model for keratoconjunctivitis sicca. Ophthalmology 99:600–604 (BS1)

International Dry Eye WorkShop (2007) Report of the International Dry Eye WorkShop. Ocul Surf 5(2):65–206

Matsumoto Y, Ohashi Y, Watanabe H, Tsubota K, Diquafosol Ophthalmic Solution Phase 2 Study Group (2012) Efficacy and safety of diquafosol ophthalmic solution in patients with dry eye syndrome: a Japanese phase 2 clinical trial. Ophthalmology 119(10):1954–1960

Rieger G (1990) Lipid-containing eye drops: a step closer to natural tears. Ophthalmologica 201:206–212

Schaumberg DA, Sullivan DA, Buring JE, Dana MR (2003) Prevalence of dry eye syndrome among US women. Am J Ophthalmol 136:318–326

Shigeyasu C, Hirano S, Akune Y, Mochizuki H, Yamada M (2013) Evaluation of the frequency of ophthalmic solution application: washout effects of topical saline application on tear components. Curr Eye Res 38:722–728

Medical Management of Dry Eye

5

Victor L. Caparas

There is no "magic bullet" in the treatment of dry eye. This is partly due to a disconnect between what patients with dry eye complain of and what doctors can observe and measure (Schein et al. 1997). It is common to see a patient who complains of significant symptoms of dry eye and yet has normal objective test results. Conversely, another patient can exhibit clinical signs of dry eye and yet be absolutely comfortable.

However, that is not to say that treatment cannot be approached scientifically. A more comprehensive understanding of the pathophysiology of dry eye has resulted in our realization that simply hydrating and lubricating the ocular surface are inadequate. Inflammation, tear composition and dynamics, and preservation of the delicate homeostasis of the ocular surface are now integral considerations in treating dry eye. While it is not yet possible to completely eliminate symptoms, we can often significantly improve the patient's condition. Despite an incomplete understanding of the pathologic processes of dry eye, we can set treatment goals and definite parameters by which to gauge success of treatment. Without reasonable guidelines, however imperfect dry eye treatment can be very frustrating.

Given our current knowledge, we now aim to return the ocular surface and tear film to its normal homeostatic state, hopefully improving the patient's ocular comfort and quality of life (or vice versa).

The following chapter attempts to briefly describe the various treatment options for dry eye that are available to the clinician as well as the rationale for each option in daily practice. It does not aim to be an exhaustive compendium of dry eye treatments but rather a practical guide that will hopefully provide the practitioner a more systematic way of approaching treatment of what can often be a confusing and frustrating condition.

5.1 Treatment Goals

Once a diagnosis of dry eye has been made, the following specific treatment goals are desirable and measurable in a general clinic setting (Table 5.1):

A good understanding of the objectives of therapy is necessary to select the proper course of action for a patient with dry eye. The 2007 DEWS Report on Management and Therapy lists the current treatments available, whose efficacy can be backed by evidence (Table 5.2) (Pflugfelder et al. 2007).

Figure 5.1 illustrates my simplified version of the dry eye cycle and the possible areas in the pathogenesis of dry eye wherein those evidence-backed treatments listed in Table 5.2 may be effective.

V.L. Caparas, MD, MPH
Department of Ophthalmology, The Medical City,
Medical Arts Tower, Suite 1912, Ortigas Avenue,
Pasig City, Metro Manila 1600, Philippines
e-mail: victor.caparas@gmail.com

C. Chan (ed.), *Dry Eye: A Practical Approach*, Essentials in Ophthalmology,
DOI 10.1007/978-3-662-44106-0_5, © Springer-Verlag Berlin Heidelberg 2015

Our currently accepted approach is to base treatment on the severity of the disease, progressively adding treatment modalities with increasing signs and symptoms (as measured by tests described earlier in this book). The 2007 Dry Eye Workshop modified the approach originally taken by the International Task Force Delphi Panel for dry eye treatment, which based treatment recommendations on disease severity (Behrens et al. 2006) (Table 5.3). [N.B. For convenience the treatment recommendations originally formulated by the ITF and modified by DEWS has been appended to the bottom of the table.]

Table 5.1 Treatment goals and their measurable parameters

Treatment goals	Tests
Relieve symptoms	Symptom questionnaire: McMonnies, OSDI
Enhance lubrication	Lid-wiper fluorescein staining
Stabilize tear film	TFBUT
Protect ocular surface cells	Ocular Protection Index
Retard evaporative tear loss	Tear film lipid layer thickness (by slit lamp)
Suppress inflammation	Oxford scheme/NEI-Industry scheme
Support meibomian gland function	Slit lamp microscopy
Maintain adequate secretion	Schirmer I, tear film meniscus (by slit lamp)

OSDI ocular surface disease index, *TFBUT* tear film break-up time

Table 5.2 Dry eye menu of treatments

Artificial tears substitutes
Gels/ointments
Moisture chamber spectacles
Anti-inflammatory agents (topical CsA and corticosteroids, omega-3 fatty acids)
Tetracyclines
Plugs
Secretagogues
Serum
Contact lenses systemic immunosuppressives
Surgery (AMT, lid surgery, tarsorrhaphy, MM and SG transplant)

Reprinted with permission. Pflugfelder et al. (2007)
AMT amniotic membrane transplantation, *MM* mucous membrane, *SG* salivary gland

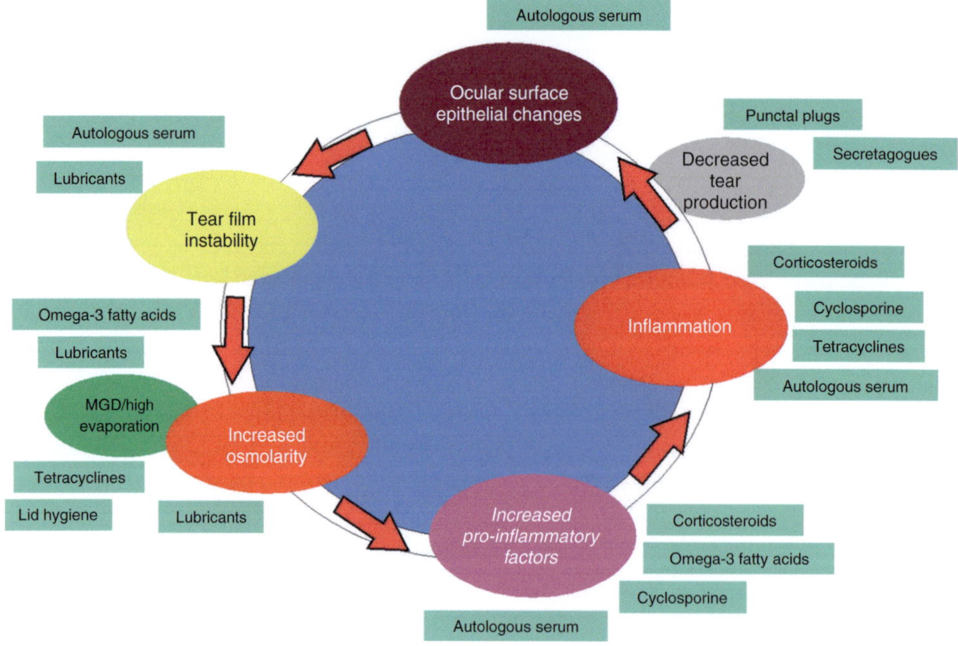

Fig. 5.1 Dry eye cycle

Table 5.3 Dry eye severity grading scheme and treatment recommendations

Dry eye severity level	1	2	3	4
Discomfort, severity, and frequency	Mild and/or episodic Occurs under environmental stress	Moderate episodic or chronic Stress or no stress	Severe frequent or constant without stress	Severe and/or disabling and constant
Visual symptoms	None or episodic mild fatigue	Annoying and/or activity-limiting episodic	Annoying chronic and/or constant limiting activity	Constant and/or possibly disabling
Conjunctival injection	None to mild	None to mild	+/−	+/++
Conjunctival staining	None to mild	Variable	Moderate to marked	Marked
Corneal staining (severity/location)	None to mild	Variable	Marked central	Severe punctate erosion
Corneal/tear signs	None to mild	Mild debris, ↓ tear meniscus	Filamentary keratitis, mucus clumping, ↑ tear debris	Filamentary keratitis, mucus clumping, ↑ tear debris, ulceration
Lid/meibomian glands	MGD variably present	MGD variably present	Frequent	Trichiasis, keratinization, symblepharon
TFBUT (s)	Variable	≤10	≤5	Immediate
Schirmer score (mm/5 min)	Variable	≤10	≤5	≤2
Treatment	Education and environmental/dietary modifications	*If level 1 treatments inadequate, add:*	*If level 2 treatments inadequate, add:*	*If level 3 treatments inadequate, add:*
	Elimination of offending systemic medications	Anti-inflammatories	Serum	Systemic anti-inflammatory agents
	Artificial tear substitutes, gels/ointments	Tetracyclines (for meibomianitis, rosacea)	Contact lenses	Surgery (lid surgery, tarsorrhaphy; mucus membrane, salivary gland, amniotic membrane transplantation)
	Eye lid therapy	Punctal plugs	Permanent punctual occlusion	
		Secretagogues		
		Moisture chamber spectacles		

Reprinted from Behrens et al. (2006)

5.2 Pharmacologic Therapy

5.2.1 Lubricants ("Artificial Tears")

Ocular lubricants are the first and, for a long time, the only "line of defense" against dry eye. All modern ocular lubricants contain electrolytes, surfactants, and viscosity agents in a hypotonic or isotonic buffered solution (Table 5.4). They vary mostly in electrolyte composition, osmolarity, viscous agent, and the presence or absence of a preservative. But while a few limited studies have tended to show the benefit to the ocular surface of certain preparations containing certain types and concentrations of electrolytes, or a certain degree of osmolarity, or greater retention of the viscous agent, there is no evidence that any agent is superior to another (Pflugfelder et al. 2007) nor is there a consensus among both physicians and patients as to the superiority of any preparation. Figure 5.2, which shows the prescribing preferences of the different types of ocular lubricants across the globe, clearly demonstrates this fact (IMS 2012).

However, there is admittedly a general consensus and considerable evidence that the use of these preparations generally does result in the amelioration of symptoms as well as improvement in objective signs (McCann et al. 2012), especially in cases of mild dry eye, thus justifying their use as a staple in dry eye medication.

Lubricants benefit dry eye patients through one or more of the following mechanisms:

1. Provides a lubricating layer between the lid-wiper edge of the palpebral conjunctiva of the upper lid and the ocular surface, i.e., relieves lid-wiper epitheliopathy (lid-wiper epitheliopathy is found in as much as 88 % of patients with symptoms – but no clinical signs – of dry eye) (Korb et al. 2010).
2. Stabilizes the tear film, decreases optical aberrations, and improves the optical quality of vision (Montés-Micó 2007).
3. May provide a "pseudo anti-inflammatory" effect, by:
    (a) Physical washing away of proinflammatory agents
    (b) Lowering tear osmolarity, through a diluting effect
    (c) Reducing the friction of lid-wiper epitheliopathy and reducing proinflammatory stress (Korb et al. 2005)
    (d) Aiding in corneal epithelial healing resulting in lower inflammation of the ocular surface (Daull et al. 2012)

> **Did you know?**
> The ocular lubricants presently available in the United States are approved based on compliance with the US Food and Drug Administration (FDA) monograph on over-the-counter (OTC) products (21 CFR 349) which provides guidelines for the inclusion of active and inactive ingredients and for solution parameters, but are not based on clinical efficacy (Pflugfelder et al. 2007).

> **Caveat**
> Despite the benefits of ocular lubricants in patients with dry eye, no preparation has been found through controlled studies to have resolved or "cured" the underlying ocular surface disease of dry eye.

Table 5.4 Ocular lubricant properties

Component/characteristic	Claimed effect/benefit
Electrolytes	Potassium: maintain corneal thickness (Green et al. 1992); increase conjunctival goblet cell density; increase corneal glycogen content (Gilbard and Rossi 1992)
	Bicarbonate: recovery of damaged epithelial barrier function; maintain normal epithelial ultrastructure; maintain mucin layer (Ubels et al. 1995)
Compatible solutes (e.g., glycerin)	Increase intracellular osmolarity, protecting against possible damage from hyperosmolar tears (Lemp 2008)
Viscosity agents	Increases residence in eye; provides patient comfort; protects damaged surface epithelium; increase tear film lipid layer
Preservatives	Protects against microbial contamination; toxic to epithelium

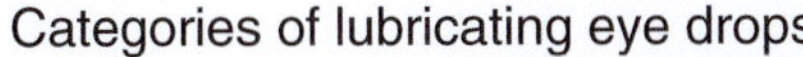

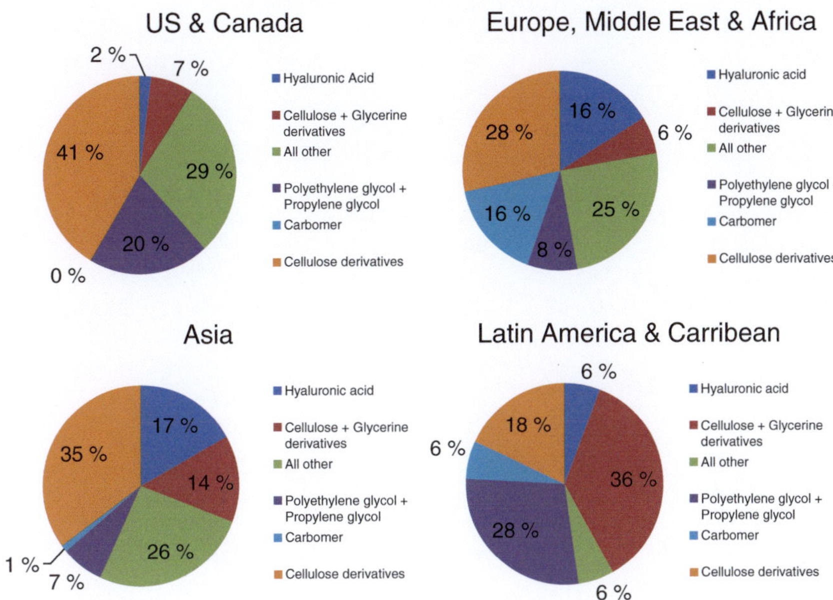

Fig. 5.2 Global ocular lubricants. The statements, findings, conclusions, views, and opinions contained and expressed in this publication are based in part on data obtained under license from the following IMS AG information service(s) (IMS MIDAS (Retail and Hospital) and OTCims (Retail Sales), FY 2012, Alcon Dry Eye Custom Market Definition, Extracted from Q4 2012 database. All Rights Reserved. The statements, findings, conclusions, views, and opinions contained and expressed herein are not necessarily those of IMS Health Incorporated or any of its affiliated or subsidiary entities)

5.2.2 Choosing a Lubricant

Often the choice of a lubricant will depend on the convenience to the patient. Will the drop stay in the eye long enough to give a sustained period of relief, or does it have to be re-instilled very frequently? This has special significance with drops containing a preservative, for which 4–6 times a day is the recommended limit (Berdy et al. 1992). Although clearly beneficial, preservative-free preparations in unit dose containers are more expensive and may be more cumbersome to use, especially for elderly patients. Preparations containing non-BAK preservatives may be better tolerated than BAK-preserved drops, although there is no evidence of lower toxicity with increased frequency of use. Lastly, increasing the viscosity of the eye drop improves retention time in the eye but results, in general, in increased blurring of vision and unsightly caking on the lids and matting of the lashes.

Ointments and gels have the advantage over solutions of increased retention time in the eye. This property allows for extended comfort for the patient. Additionally, ointments do not support bacterial growth and therefore need not contain preservatives. However, owing to their higher viscosity, ointments and gels significantly interfere with visual function and as a result are usually reserved for severe cases and nighttime use.

Practical Questions for Choosing a Lubricant
1. Does the medication relieve symptoms?
2. Does the preparation stay in the eye long enough to protect the ocular surface and provide comfort?
3. How often will it be instilled in the eye daily?
4. Does it contain a preservative, and if it does, which preservative?
5. Does it impair visual function or cause unsightly caking on the lids and lashes?

Table 5.5 Gross residence time data (time, in min, for signal to regain baseline)

Subject	Saline 1	0.3 % PG	CMC 0.5 %	CMC 1.0 %	Oil emulsion	HPMC 0.3 % gel	HPMC 0.3 % solution	Saline 2
1	24	44	30	38	NT[a]	26	NT	26
2	21	72 plus[b]	34 plus	72 plus[b]	NT	44	NT	6.6
3	22	38	26	24	NT	18	NT	7.53
4	22.2	47	28.6	86	NT	54	NT	40
5	10.5	32	14	50	NT	24	NT	22
6	22.7	30	12	30	18	NT	31	19.5
7	14.1	16.5	14.5	36	7.4	NT	16.2	12.2
8	14	54.4	40	40	20	NT	28.4	26
9	6.1	18.7	20	16.2	14	NT	20	14.5
10	14.3	14	12	18	12	NT	13.9	16
11	29.8	36	18	46	32	NT	26	18
12	18.3	28	20	36	12	NT	14	12
13	36	55.5	20	54	19	NT	54	12
14	20	40	22	48	28	NT	24	20
15	14	22	24	24	26	NT	26	16
16	16	32	24	34.4	10	NT	16	14
Mean	19.07	36.25	22.44	40.79	18.03	33.2	24.49	17.64
SD	7.4	15.7	7.9	18.7	7.9	15.1	11.5	8.2

Reprinted with permission: Paugh et al. (2008)
[a]NT means formulation was not tested in this subject
[b]Subject had to leave before return to baseline; thus endpoint is conservative

Despite lacking clear evidence supporting superior efficacy of one lubricant preparation over another, many clinicians do have certain preferences based on their assessment of the patient's dry eye condition. They make their choice of lubricant based on the previously mentioned practical considerations, patient preference, and their understanding, based on the limited evidence, of the strengths and purported features of a certain preparation. For example, recent reports have shown that drops containing oil in emulsion, by improving the lipid layer of the tear film, appear to perform better than conventional lubricants HPMC and sodium hyaluronate in evaporative dry eye (McCann et al. 2012). Given the current interest in the role of meibomian gland dysfunction in dry eye, many clinicians prefer to prescribe such oil-based preparations to their patients with MGD and dry eye.

Tables 5.5 and 5.6 below illustrate the ocular residence time and the lubricity (expressed as coefficient of friction) of various substances used in popular commercial preparations (Paugh et al. 2008; Meyer et al. 2007).

Table 5.6 Comparison of post-rinse (stage IV) coefficients of friction (tissue-on-tissue experiments)

Formulation	Final average coefficient for each of 3 replicate experiments	Average (SD)
Saline control	0.384, 0.263, 0.223	0.290 (0.068)
HPMC solution	0.109, 0.135, 0.156	0.133 (0.019)
CMC solution	0.252, 0.453, 0.291	0.332 (0.087)
Glycerin emulsion	0.265, 0.156, 0.174	0.198 (0.048)
SYS 1	0.051, 0.057, 0.047	0.052 (0.004)
SYS 2	0.041, 0.017, 0.041	0.033 (0.011)
SYS 3	0.047, 0.122, 0.007	0.059 (0.048)

Reprinted with permission: Meyer et al. (2007)

The longer an instilled eye drop stays in the eye, the longer the protection and comfort. The lower the coefficient of friction, the greater the lubricity, resulting in less friction between palpebral conjunctiva and the ocular surface.

Again, while there is no firm evidence that one preparation is superior to the other, knowledge of the physical characteristics which influence the behavior in the eye of these substances aids practitioners in making a more systematic and scientific choice of ocular lubricant.

My Personal Preferences
1. For mainly symptomatic patients with little or no objective signs of dry eye and whose needs do not require more than 3–4 times application daily, I prefer to use low-viscosity solutions (to avoid blurring) without a preservative or a mild, non-BAK preservative. Additionally, many of these patients suffer from lid-wiper epitheliopathy and benefit from agents with high lubricity (low coefficient of friction).
2. For patients with moderate symptoms and with ocular surface staining, my preference is for solutions with low viscosity but with higher ocular retention, such as the liquid polyols (especially when linked with a gelling agent like HP-Guar) or sodium hyaluronate. The longer retention time and "bandage effect" of these agents protect and allow healing of the damaged epithelium. Non-preserved preparations are desirable.
3. Dry eye with MGD requires oil-based emulsions to augment the lipid layer of the tear film and reduce evaporation.
4. With more severe keratopathy, those preparations with high ocular retention and high colloidal osmolality (for deturgescent effect on damaged epithelial cells) are desirable. Gels and ointments may be necessary for severe cases.

5.3 Anti-inflammatory Therapy

The application of anti-inflammatory therapy (Table 5.7) in cases of dry eye is based on the central role played by inflammation in the initiation and propagation of dry eye. Good clinical evidence supports the efficacy of anti-inflammatory eye drops in improving severity of symptoms and decreasing corneal staining in moderate to severe dry eye, when compared to ocular lubricant therapy *alone*.

5.3.1 Corticosteroids

Topical corticosteroids are a valuable adjunct to therapy. They are used to disrupt the vicious cycle of inflammation and epithelial damage. The immediate value to the practitioner is that they often afford the patient quick relief from their discomfort. Of course, the many well-known side effects of corticosteroids, of which glaucoma is most notable, dictate short- rather than long-term use. Topical corticosteroids with lower intraocular activity and lower risk to increasing intraocular pressure (so-called "soft steroids"), such as fluorometholone and loteprednol, should be considered if long-term anti-inflammatory therapy is needed. Cyclosporine is a significant addition to our arsenal in that it offers immunomodulatory and anti-inflammatory actions, without the side effects of corticosteroids.

5.3.2 Cyclosporine

T cells appear to play a significant role in the pathogenesis of dry eye. Involved exocrine

Table 5.7 Anti-inflammatory agents for dry eye treatment

Agent	Mechanism
Corticosteroids	Inhibit production of proinflammatory cytokines GM-CSF, IL-6, IL-8, MCP-3, and RANTES (Djalilian et al. 2006) decrease expression of ICAM system (Lu et al. 2005)
Cyclosporine	Inhibits T-cell activity, selectively inhibiting release of cytokines like IL-1 (Matsuda and Koyasu 2000; Kunert et al. 2000) Significantly reduced conjunctival epithelial apoptosis and protected against goblet cell loss in experimental murine dry eye (Strong et al. 2005)
Tetracyclines	Decrease activity of collagenase, phospholipase A2, and matrix metalloproteinases; decrease production of IL-1 and TNF-α (Solomon et al. 2000) inhibit Staphylococcal exotoxin-induced cytokines (Krakauer and Buckley 2003)
Autologous serum	May inhibit inflammatory cytokines, e.g., IL-1 and TNF-α; inhibit matrix metalloproteinases (Liou 2001; Tsubota et al. 1999a, b)
Omega-3 fatty acids	Inhibit synthesis of proinflammatory lipid mediators PGE2, LBT4; block production of IL-1 and TNF-α (James et al. 2000; Endres et al. 1989)

TNF tumor necrosis factor, *ICAM* intercellular adhesion molecule, *IL-1* interleukin-1, *PGE2* prostaglandin E2, *LBT4* leukotriene B4

tissues in Sjogren's syndrome are infiltrated with lymphocytes, monocytes, and plasma cells (Carsons 2001). The conjunctiva of both Sjogren's and non-Sjogren's keratoconjunctivitis sicca is infiltrated by T cells (Pflugfelder et al. 1990). Infiltration of CD4+ T was accompanied by increased expression of IFN-gamma, goblet cell loss, and conjunctival metaplasia (De Paiva et al. 2007).

Studies have shown that cyclosporine is capable of addressing the causes of dry eye rather than being merely palliative as, for example, lubricants are. Cyclosporine has been demonstrated to reduce conjunctival IL-6 levels (Turner et al. 2000), decrease activated lymphocytes in conjunctiva (Kunert et al. 2000), reduce conjunctival inflammatory and apoptotic markers (Brignole et al. 2001), and increase conjunctival goblet cell numbers (Kunert et al. 2002). Clinically, in two 6-month, multicenter, randomized, double-blind, vehicle-controlled phase 3 trials, cyclosporine was significantly more effective than vehicle in improving two objective outcomes (corneal fluorescein staining and Schirmer's with anesthesia) and three subjective outcomes (blurred vision, need for artificial tears, and physician's evaluation of global response). It is interesting to note that both cyclosporine alone and vehicle alone significantly decreased symptoms and objective signs compared with baseline, and there were no between-group differences in conjunctival staining, Schirmer test without anesthesia, or symptoms other than blurred vision (Sall et al. 2000). Additionally, continued use of cyclosporine for up to 3 years resulted only in minimal ocular adverse events and risk for systemic toxicity (Sall et al. 2000; Barber et al. 2005; Small et al. 2002). Based on this evidence, cyclosporine is currently the only pharmacologic agent approved by the US FDA for the treatment of dry eye.

Tips in Using Cyclosporine
1. Cyclosporine is no panacea for dry eye. It works best in cases were inflammation is a significant component of the disease. For a quicker response, a short, 1–2-week course of topical corticosteroids may be instituted at the same time cyclosporine is started.
2. Its onset of action is slow, and that patience should be advised in case improvement in symptoms and signs are not immediately forthcoming. The recommended duration of treatment is 6 months.
3. The most common adverse events are stinging and redness, which in most cases do not warrant or have led to cessation of cyclosporine.

5.3.3   Tetracycline Derivatives

The tetracycline derivatives (Table 5.8) are used in the therapy of dry eye mainly for their anti-inflammatory and lipid-regulating roles in the treatment of MGD and rosacea. With the exception of minocycline, at currently accepted dosages, the antimicrobial actions of tetracycline derivatives are limited.

> **Tips in Using Tetracyclines**
> 1. Doxycycline and minocycline achieve higher tissue concentrations compared to tetracycline and oxytetracycline, a characteristic which may be explained by their higher lipophilicity (Hoeprich and Warshauer 1974). This allows for higher activity at lower concentrations, increasing safety.
> 2. At 100 mg a day, minocycline differs from other derivatives by achieving levels that not only inhibit lipase production but reduce lid flora but as well (Ta et al. 2003).

> 3. The longer the duration of intake, the higher the risk for side effects and complications. A 3-month course of minocycline has been shown to be efficacious up to 3 months following cessation of therapy (Aronowicz et al. 2006).

5.3.4   Azithromycin

Azithromycin is a macrolide antibiotic that has been shown to suppress inflammatory cytokines (TNF-α, IL-1β) and chemokines (IL-8, RANTES, and matrix metalloproteinases MMP-1, MMP-3, and MMP-9) by blocking nuclear factor-κB activation in human corneal epithelial cells (Li et al. 2010). Consequently it has been used to treat ocular surface infections and MGD. In an open-label study, azithromycin with warm lid compresses was compared to lid compresses alone. The azithromycin group showed significant improvements in meibomian gland plugging, quality of meibomian gland secretions, and eyelid redness after a 12-day treatment period (Luchs 2008). In a more recent prospective open-label study,

Table 5.8   Tetracycline derivatives and presumed actions

Agent	Mechanism of action in dry eye	Dosage
Tetracycline derivatives, in general	Decrease the activity of collagenase, phospholipase A$_2$, and several matrix metalloproteinases	250 mg once to 4 times a day
	Decrease the production of IL-1α and TNF-α in corneal epithelium (Solomon et al. 2000)	
	Inhibit staphylococcal exotoxin-induced cytokines and chemokines (Krakauer and Buckley 2003; Dougherty et al. 1991)	
	Inhibit matrix metalloproteinase expression (Stone and Chodosh 2004)	
	Inhibit angiogenesis (Tamargo et al. 1991)	
Doxycycline	Decreases gelatinolytic activity in the ocular surface epithelia, as well as decreases levels of MMP-9 mRNA transcripts, and prevents experimental dry eye-induced increase in IL-1 and TNF-α (De Paiva et al. 2006)	50–100 mg once or twice a day
Minocycline	Attenuate TNF-α, IL-1β, IL-8, and IL-6 production (Ledeboer et al. 2005)	
	Suppressive effects on inflammatory cells, T lymphocytes, and monocytes, resulting in inhibitory effect on TNF-α, MMP-9, and IFN-γ production (Kloppenburg et al. 1996)	
	Changes fatty acid composition of meibum (Souchier et al. 2008)	

once-daily topical therapy for 4 weeks with azithromycin was shown to have relieved signs and symptoms of MGD and restored the lipid properties of the meibomian gland secretion toward normal (Foulks et al. 2010). Current recommendation for use of azithromycin is to reserve its use until it is proven that erythromycin is not effective. This is due to the significant difference in cost. When used, it is started as a twice daily application, directly to the lashes, for 2 days and a once-daily application for the next 28 days (Veldman and Colby 2011). While promising, topical azithromycin is a relatively new product and still unavailable to most clinicians outside the United States. More experience and investigations are definitely needed to confirm its usefulness.

5.3.5 Omega-3 Fatty Acids

When dietary intake of omega-6 and omega-3 fatty acids was studied, as part of the Women's Health Study, a significantly increased risk of dry eye syndrome was observed in women consuming a higher ratio of omega-6 to omega-3 fatty acids (Miljanovic et al. 2005). The average Western diet is said to have 20–25 times more omega-6 than omega-3 (Pflugfelder et al. 2007). Significantly lower levels of inflammatory mediators IL IL-1β, IL6, and IL10 in tears were significantly lower in the group of non-severe dry eye subjects receiving daily antioxidant and omega-3 fatty acid supplements (DHA 350 mg, EPA 42.5 mg, DPA 30 mg). Additionally, subjective symptoms of dry eye significantly improved in this same group compared to the group not receiving dietary supplements (Pinazo-Durán et al. 2013). However, despite widespread acceptance by practitioners of the benefits of omega-3 fatty acid supplementation, current data related to its beneficial use in dry eye remains unclear. A large multicenter, randomized, clinical trial is needed to clarify its role.

5.3.6 Autologous Serum

Serum contains several anti-inflammatory factors that may inhibit the elaboration of mediators of inflammation on the ocular surface (Liou 2001) which may explain partly its ability to improve signs and symptoms in patients with dry eye.

Practical Tips for Anti-inflammatory Treatment

1. For short-term or episodic inflammation, I practice a "pulsed" dosing of a topical corticosteroid, 2–3 times a day, for a maximum of 2 weeks. My preference is for "soft" corticosteroid drops such as fluorometholone and loteprednol to minimize the risk of side effects, especially increased intraocular pressure.
2. For long-term or chronic causes of inflammation, I switch to cyclosporine twice a day.
3. In addition to this, at least 450 mg of omega-3 fatty acids supplement is added (Pinazo-Durán et al. 2013).
4. MGD is frequently present in these long-term cases, and I prescribe daily doxycycline for as long as 3 months at a time. I prescribe a single dose of 100 mg daily but only because it is the lowest concentration available in the market in which I practice. Different markets have different preparations. Use of as low as 20 mg twice a day has been shown to be effective (Yoo et al. 2005).
5. Where cost to the patient is an issue, autologous serum in lieu of cyclosporine and non-preserved lubricants may be a good alternative.

5.4 Autologous Serum

The use of autologous serum (Table 5.9) has been found to significantly improve symptoms and conjunctival and corneal staining and TBUT scores in cases of severe dry eye. Other studies report successful use in the treatment of cases of persistent epithelial defects, superior limbic keratoconjunctivitis, and graft-versus-host disease with dry eye (Tsubota et al. 1999a, b; Goto et al. 2001; Ogawa et al. 2003. It has also been

Table 5.9 Serum components and presumed benefit to ocular surface

Serum component	Presumed effect on ocular surface
Retinoic acid	Upregulates MUC-4 and MUC-16 (Hori et al. 2004)
EGF	Anti-apoptotic property, aids in healing epithelium (Collins et al. 1994)
TGF-β	Responsible fibroblast activation in wound healing (Collins et al. 1994)
FGF	Stimulates corneal stromal wound healing (Fredj-Reygrobellet et al. 1987)
Fibronectin	Provides temporary matrix for cell migration (Phan et al. 1987)
Vitamin A	Promotes epithelial differentiation, decreases ocular surface metaplasia (Tsubota et al. 1999a, b)
Vitamin E	Prevent keratocyte apoptosis (Bilgihan et al. 2001)
HGF	Modulates corneal epithelial cell proliferation (Chandrasekher et al. 2001)
PDGF	Modulate corneal fibroblasts' proliferation and increase migration during homeostasis and wound healing (Andresen et al. 1997)

MUC mucin, *EGF* epidermal growth factor, *TGF-β* transforming growth factor-beta, *FGF* fibroblast growth factor, *HGF* human growth factor, *PDGF* platelet-derived growth factor

shown that concomitant use with a silicon contact lens can be effective in treating persistent epithelial defects (Choi and Chung 2011).

While many reports describe generally successful treatments, the efficacy of autologous serum varies significantly. Liu et al. hypothesized that different processes produced varying concentrations of serum components and attempted to standardize the production process of serum. This resulted in the extraction and retention of an "optimal" amount of epitheliotropic factors in serum (Liu et al. 2005). We have adopted this process at our center:

> **"Optimized" Production Process of Autologous Serum (Liu)**
> 1. Procure 100 ml of blood by venipuncture, and store in sterile containers.
> 2. Perform routine virology testing: HbsAg (antibodies to HCV, HIV I and II) and syphilis (HCV NAT).
> 3. Leave containers upright for 2 h in room temperature (18–25 °C).
> 4. Centrifuge at 3,000 × g for 15 min.
> 5. Transfer supernatant (average volume, 30–35 ml) into 50 ml disposable syringes in laminar flow hood.
> 6. Dilute serum 1:4 with BSS.
> 7. Aliquot into sterile dropper bottles after gentle shaking.
> 8. Label each bottle with name and date of birth of patient and date of production of serum.
> 9. Store at −20 °C for maximum of 3 months.
> 10. Apply drops 8× daily.
> 11. Store open bottle at +4 °C.
> 12. Discard open bottle after 16 h of use.

5.5 Nonpharmacologic Treatment

5.5.1 Punctal Plugs

Punctal plugs are widely acknowledged to provide symptomatic improvement and to improve objective signs from baseline measures, yet under more stringent scrutiny, only a few studies demonstrate a benefit of punctal plugs over the comparison intervention. A systematic review published in 2010 showed a relative scarcity of controlled clinical trials assessing the efficacy of punctal occlusion therapy in dry eye (Ervin et al. 2010). More recently, however, more sensitive tests such as functional visual acuity testing, designed to establish an accurate representation of the effects of dry eye treatments on visual function (Torkildsen 2009), have been used to assess the comparative efficacies of different dry eye treatments, including the use of punctal plugs. For example, it was shown that punctal occlusion of both upper and lower puncta was effective for patients with post-LASIK dry eye that could not be controlled by artificial tears alone. Not only were symptoms and tear function improved but also the quality of vision, as measured by functional visual acuity (Yung et al. 2012). FVA was also used to differentiate the effects of plugging either the lower or upper punctum, both of which resulted in significant improvement of vital staining scores and TBUT times. However, functional visual acuity values significantly improved only in eyes receiving upper punctal plug occlusion (Kaido et al. 2012).

> **Practical Tips in Using Punctal Plugs**
> 1. Permanent silicone plugs have not been shown to be superior in efficacy to temporary collagen plugs for short-term use (Ervin et al. 2010). Where cost is an issue, the less expensive collagen plugs are more accessible to patients who need them.
> 2. The DEWS recommendation is to use punctal plugs as early as dry eye severity level 2 when there exists, among other parameters, moderate discomfort and mild visual function impairment.
> 3. It is important to use punctal plugs until after anti-inflammatory therapy has been instituted and has reduced the expression of proinflammatory cyto- and chemokines. Otherwise, these will continue to circulate in conjunctival sac and perpetuate the inflammation. The same logic applies to the presence of chronic ocular surface or lid infection.
> 4. Similarly, the residence time of any topical medication instilled in the conjunctival sac may be extended by punctal occlusion. As a result, such medication's effect may be potentiated (Zimmerman et al. 1984) with possible consequences on dosing and patient compliance (Roberts et al. 2007).

5.5.2 Environmental and Lifestyle Modification

Patient education is often overlooked in the treatment of dry eye. A significant number of a person's daily activities have the capacity to

Table 5.10 Lifestyle changes

Lifestyle modifications	Reduce or eliminate offending systemic medications, e.g., antihistamines, antidepressants, diuretics, beta-blockers
	Reduce or eliminate use of ocular vasoconstrictors
	Instruct on proper use/lubrication of contact lenses
	Instruct on the harmful effects of preservatives in eye drops, and to avoid, if possible
	Reduction/cessation of smoking, alcohol consumption
	Recommend daily eye lid hygiene: warm lid compresses (for MGD and chronic blepharitis)
Environmental modifications	Avoid low humidity, high-temperature environments
	Avoid windy, drafty places/instruct on protective eyewear
	Position computer screen below eye level
	Take regular breaks from computer work ("20-20 Rule": 20 min working at computer; 20 s focus away from screen)
Dietary modifications	Instruct on adequate vitamin A intake
	Recommend increase omega-3 essential fatty acids
	Decrease omega-6 essential fatty acids
	Recommend increase linoleic and gamma-linolenic fatty acids
	Encourage proper hydration
	Control diabetes/sugar intake

aggravate one's dry eye condition. Computer use, time spent in windy environments, driving, and reading have all been implicated (Iyer et al. 2012). It is important to note that mild degrees of dry eye can be treated successfully with lifestyle modification (Table 5.10) and a minimum of medication (Behrens et al. 2006).

While there has been no definitive study measuring the impact of lifestyle and environmental changes on the dry eye condition, the potential benefit of most of these changes is universally accepted, yet often overlooked in the education of the dry eye patient.

5.6 Summary

Our understanding of the etiology and mechanism of dry eye has grown exponentially in a matter of a few years. Regrettably, much of this new data has not translated into improving the tools clinicians need in alleviating the suffering of their patients. While waiting for new treatments which address the new knowledge to be developed, the current chapter offers an interim approach, based on rationalizing the treatment of dry eye by the clinician by stating clear objectives for which a certain agent can be applied and its efficacy measured. It is therefore of prime importance to understand the benefit and limitations that each therapeutic agent brings.

Unfortunately, in the clinic setting, the multitude of commercial products marketed for the "treatment of dry eye" can confuse both doctors and patients alike. The case of ocular lubricants, which by far is the most accessible and most prescribed agent, is a prime example. Having an updated understanding of dry eye syndrome, in particular, the importance of instability of the tear film, is necessary for a more rational basis for choice of lubricants. For most preparations, the physical properties of the lubricant – viscosity, elasticity, and lubricity – are manipulated to decrease lid-to-ocular surface friction and increase retention time in the eye to provide surface protection and allow underlying damaged epithelium to heal, thus often resulting in symptom relief. However, it is clear that these lubricants have little or no effect on currently held beliefs of the mechanism of dry eye, such as inflammation. Therefore to be able to successfully treat dry eye, the clinicians should be able to recognize certain specific treatment objectives for which their arsenal should extend, beyond lubricants.

Addressing inflammation, which can be readily assessed clinically, is a key treatment goal. As the role of inflammation is further clarified, an ever-increasing variety of treatment agents is now available to the clinician. The appropriate use of these agents results in improvement of signs and symptoms unattainable by lubricants alone. However, the risks and additional costs of utilizing these agents demand a deeper understanding on the timing and duration of their use.

It is clear also that as voluminous as our current understanding is of the development of dry eye, much needs to be elucidated of other factors such as environmental influences. Here, relatively little attention has been given by both researchers and clinicians alike, and this remains to be a gaping hole in our knowledge.

It should be reiterated that a completely dependable treatment for dry eye does not yet exist. In the meantime, using a rational, directed approach based on current knowledge and treatment modalities, clinicians can achieve consistent, albeit qualified, success in alleviating the suffering of their dry eye patients.

Compliance with Ethical Requirements Informed consent and animal studies disclosures are not applicable to this review.

I have received speaker's honoraria from Alcon and Allergan. I do not own any stock in either company.

References

Andresen JL, Ledet T, Ehlers N (1997) Keratocyte migration and peptide growth factors: the effect of PDGF, bFGF, EGF, IGF-I, aFGF and TGF-beta on human keratocyte migration in a collagen gel. Curr Eye Res 16:605–613

Aronowicz JD, Shine WE, Oral D et al (2006) Short term oral minocyclinetreatment of meibomianitis. Br J Ophthalmol 90:856–860

Barber LD, Pflugfelder SC, Tauber J, Foulks GN (2005) Phase III safety evaluation of cyclosporine 0.1% ophthalmic emulsion administered twice daily to dry eye disease patients for up to 3 years. Ophthalmology 112:1790–1794

Behrens A, Doyle JJ, Stern L et al (2006) Dysfunctional tear syndrome. A Delphi approach to treatment recommendations. Cornea 25:90–97

Berdy GJ, Abelson MB, Smith LM, George MA (1992) Preservative-free artificial tear preparations: assessment of corneal epithelial toxic effects. Arch Ophthalmol 110:528–532

Bilgihan K, Adiguzel U, Sezer C, Akyol G, Hasanreisoglu B (2001) Effects of topical vitamin E on keratocyte apoptosis after traditional photorefractive keratectomy. Ophthalmologica 215:192–196

Brignole F, Pisella PJ, De Saint Jean M, Goldschild M, Goguel A, Baudouin C (2001) Flow cytometric analysis of inflammatory markers in KCS: 6-month treatment with topical cyclosporin A. Invest Ophthalmol Vis Sci 42:90–95

Carsons S (2001) A review and update of Sjögren's syndrome: manifestations, diagnosis, and treatment. Am J Manag Care 7(14 Suppl):S433–S443

Chandrasekher G, Kakazu AH, Bazan HE (2001) HGF- and KGF-induced activation of PI-3K/p70 s6 kinase pathway in corneal epithelial cells: its relevance in wound healing. Exp Eye Res 73:191–202

Choi JA, Chung SH (2011) Combined application of autologous serum eye drops and silicone hydrogel lenses for the treatment of persistent epithelial defects. Eye Contact Lens 37(6):370–373

Collins MK, Perkins GR, Rodriguez Tarduchy G et al (1994) Growth factors as survival factors: regulation of apoptosis. Bioessays 16:133–138

Daull P, Feraille L, Elena P, Baudouin C, Garrigue JS (2012) Comparison of the anti-inflammatory effects of artificial tears in a rat model of corneal scraping. Acta Ophthalmologica 90:0. doi:10.1111/j.1755-3768.2012.4446.x

De Paiva CS, Corrales RM, Villarreal AL, Farley WJ, Li DQ, Stern ME et al (2006) Corticosteroid and doxycycline suppress MMP-9 and inflammatory cytokine expression, MAPK activation in the corneal epithelium in experimental dry eye. Exp Eye Res 83:526–535

De Paiva CS, Villarreal AL, Corrales RM, Rahman HT, Chang VY, Farley WJ et al (2007) Dry eye-induced conjunctival epithelial squamous metaplasia is modulated by interferon-gamma. Invest Ophthalmol Vis Sci 48(6):2553–2560

Djalilian AR, Nagineni CN, Mahesh SP, Smith JA, Nussenblatt RB, Hooks JJ (2006) Inhibition of inflammatory cytokine production in human corneal cells by dexamethasone, but not cyclosporin. Cornea 25(6):709–714

Dougherty JM, Mcculley JP, Silvany RE et al (1991) The role of tetracycline in chronic blepharitis. Invest Ophthalmol Vis Sci 32:2970–2975

Endres S, Ghorbani R, Kelley VE, Georgilis K, Lonnemann G, van der Meer JW et al (1989) The effect of dietary supplementation with omega-3 polyunsaturated fatty acids on the synthesis of interleukin-1 and tumor necrosis factor by mononuclear cells. N Engl J Med 320(5):265–271

Ervin AM, Wojciechowski R, Schein O (2010) Punctal occlusion for dry eye syndrome. Cochrane Database Syst Rev (9):CD006775

Foulks GN, Borchman D, Yappert M, Kim SH, McKay JW (2010) Topical azithromycin therapy for meibomian gland dysfunction: clinical response and lipid alterations. Cornea 29(7):781–788

Fredj-Reygrobellet D, Plouet J, Delayre T et al (1987) Effects of aFGF and bFGF on wound healing in rabbit corneas. Curr Eye Res 6:1205–1209

Gilbard JP, Rossi SR (1992) An electrolyte-based solution that increases corneal glycogen and conjunctival goblet-cell density in a rabbit model for keratoconjunctivitis sicca. Ophthalmology 99:600–604

Goto E, Shimmura S, Shimazaki J et al (2001) Treatment of superior limbic keratoconjunctivitis by application of autologous serum. Cornea 20:807–810

Green K, MacKeen DL, Slagle T, Cheeks L (1992) Tear potassium contributes to maintenance of corneal thickness. Ophthalmic Res 24:99–102

Hoeprich PD, Warshauer DM (1974) Entry of four tetracyclines into saliva and tears. Antimicrob Agents Chemother 5:330–336

Hori Y, Spurr-Michaud S, Russo CL, Argüeso P, Gipson IK (2004) Differential regulation of membrane-associated mucins in the human ocular surface epithelium. Invest Ophthalmol Vis Sci 45(1):114–122

IMS MIDAS (Retail and Hospital) and OTCims (Retail Sales), FY 2012, Alcon Dry Eye Custom Market Definition, Extracted from Q4 2012 database

Iyer JV, Lee SY, Tong L (2012) The dry eye disease activity log study. ScientificWorldJournal 2012:589875. doi:10.1100/2012/589875. Epub 2012 Oct 24

James MJ, Gibson RA, Cleland LG (2000) Dietary polyunsaturated fatty acids and inflammatory mediator production. Am J Clin Nutr 71(1 Suppl):343S–348S

Kaido M, Ishida R, Dogru M, Tsubota K (2012) Visual function changes after punctal occlusion with the treatment of short BUT type of dry eye. Cornea 31(9):1009–1013

Kloppenburg M, Brinkman BM, de Rooij-Dijk HH, Miltenburg AM, Daha MR, Breedveld FC, Dijkmans BA, Verweij C (1996) The tetracycline derivative minocycline differentially affects cytokine production by monocytes and T lymphocytes. Antimicrob Agents Chemother 40(4):934–940

Korb DR, Herman JP, Greiner JV et al (2005) Lid wiper epitheliopathy and dry eye symptoms. Eye Contact Lens 31(1):2–8

Korb DR, Herman JP, Blackie CA, Scaffidi RC, Greiner JV, Exford JM, Finnemore VM (2010) Prevalence of lid wiper epitheliopathy in subjects with dry eye signs and symptoms. Cornea 29(4):377–383. doi:10.1097/ICO.0b013e3181ba0cb2

Krakauer T, Buckley M (2003) Doxycycline is anti-inflammatory and inhibits staphylococcal exotoxin-induced cytokines and chemokines. Antimicrob Agents Chemother 47(11):3630–3633

Kunert KS, Tisdale AS, Stern ME, Smith JA, Gipson IK (2000) Analysis of topical cyclosporine treatment of patients with dry eye syndrome: effect on conjunctival lymphocytes. Arch Ophthalmol 118:1489–1496

Kunert KS, Tisdale AS, Gipson IK (2002) Goblet cell numbers and epithelial proliferation in the conjunctiva of patients with dry eye syndrome treated with cyclosporine. Arch Ophthalmol 120:330–337

Ledeboer A, Sloane EM, Milligan ED, Frank MG, Mahony JH, Maier SF, Watkins LR (2005) Minocycline attenuates mechanical allodynia and proinflammatory cytokine expression in rat models of pain facilitation. Pain 115(1–2):71–83

Lemp MA (2008) Management of dry eye. Am J Manag Care 14:S088–S101, Accessed March 11, 2013

Li DQ, Zhou N, Zhang L, Ma P, Pflugfelder SC (2010) Suppressive effects of azithromycin on zymocin-induced production of proinflammatory mediators by human corneal epithelial cells. Invest Ophthalmol Vis Sci 51(11):5623–5629

Liou LB (2001) Serum and in vivo production of IL-1 receptor antagonist correlate with C-reactive protein levels in newly diagnosed, untreated lupus patients. Clin Exp Rheumatol 19:515–523

Liu L, Hartwig D, Harloff S, Herminghaus P, Wedel T, Geerling G (2005) An optimised protocol for the production of autologous serum eyedrops. Graefes Arch Clin Exp Ophthalmol 243(7): 706–714

Lu Y, Fukuda K, Nakamura Y, Kimura K, Kumagai N, Nishida T (2005) Inhibitory effect of triptolide on chemokine expression induced by proinflammatory cytokines in human corneal fibroblasts. Invest Ophthalmol Vis Sci 46(7):2346–2352

Luchs J (2008) Efficacy of topical azithromycin ophthalmic solution 1% in the treatment of posterior blepharitis. Adv Ther 25:858–870

Matsuda S, Koyasu S (2000) Mechanisms of action of cyclosporine. Immunopharmacology 47(2–3):119–125

McCann LC, Tomlinson A, Pearce EI, Papa V (2012) Effectiveness of artificial tears in the management of evaporative dry eye. Cornea 31(1):1–5. doi:10.1097/ICO.0b013e31821b71e6

Meyer AE, Baier RE, Chen H, Chowhan M (2007) Differential tissue-on-tissue lubrication by ophthalmic formulations. J Biomed Mater Res B Appl Biomater 82B:74–88

Miljanovic B, Trivedi KA, Dana MR, Gilbard JP, Buring JE, Schaumberg DA (2005) Relation between dietary n-3 and n-6 fatty acids and clinically diagnosed dry eye syndrome in women. Am J Clin Nutr 82(4): 887–893

Montés-Micó R (2007) Role of the tear film in the optical quality of the human eye. J Cataract Refract Surg 33(9):1631–1635

Ogawa Y, Okamoto S, Mori T et al (2003) Autologous serum eye drops for the treatment of severe dry eye in patients with chronic graft-versus-host disease. Bone Marrow Transplant 31:579–583

Paugh JR, Nguyen AL, Ketelson HA, Christensen MT, Meadows DL (2008) Precorneal residence time of artificial tears measured in dry eye subjects. Optom Vis Sci 85:725–731

Pflugfelder SC, Huang AJ, Feuer W, Chuchovski PT, Pereira IC, Tseng SC (1990) Conjunctival cytologic features of primary Sjögren's syndrome. Ophthalmology 97(8):985–991

Pflugfelder SC, Gerd Geerling G, Shigero Kinoshita S, Lemp MA, McCulley J, Nelson D, Novack GN, Shimazaki J, Wilson C (2007) Management and therapy of dry eye disease: report of the Management and Therapy Subcommittee of the International Dry Eye WorkShop (2007). Ocul Surf 5(2):163–178

Phan TM, Foster CS, BoruchoV SA et al (1987) Topical fibronectin in the treatment of persistent corneal epithelial defects and trophic ulcers. Am J Ophthalmol 104:494–501

Pinazo-Durán MD, Galbis-Estrada C, Pons-Vázquez S, Cantú-Dibildox J, Marco-Ramírez C, Benítez-Del-Castillo J (2013) Effects of a nutraceutical formulation based on the combination of antioxidants and ?-3 essential fatty acids in the expression of inflammation and immune response mediators in tears from patients with dry eye disorders. Clin Interv Aging 8:139–148

Roberts CW, Carniglia PE, Brazzo BG (2007) Comparison of topical cyclosporine, punctal occlusion, and a combination for the treatment of dry eye. Cornea 26(7):805–809

Sall K, Stevenson OD, Mundorf TK, Reis BL (2000) Two multi- center, randomized studies of the efficacy and safety of cyclosporine ophthalmic emulsion in moderate to severe dry eye disease. CsA Phase 3 Study Group. Ophthalmology 107:631–639

Schein OD, Tielsch JM, Munõz B, Bandeen-Roche K, West S (1997) Relation between signs and symptoms of dry eye in the elderly. A population-based perspective. Ophthalmology 104(9):1395–1401

Small DS, Acheampong A, Reis B, Stern K, Stewart W, Berdy G, Epstein R, Foerster R, Forstot L, Tang-Liu DD (2002) Blood concentrations of cyclosporin A during long-term treatment with cyclosporin A ophthalmic emulsions in patients with moderate to severe dry eye disease. J Ocul Pharmacol Ther 18:411–418

Solomon A, Rosenblatt M, Li DQ, Liu Z, Monroy D, Ji Z et al (2000) Doxycycline inhibition of interleukin-1 in the corneal epithelium. Invest Ophthalmol Vis Sci 41(9):2544–2557

Souchier M, Joffre C, Grégoire S, Bretillon L, Muselier A, Acar N, Beynat J, Bron A, D'Athis P, Creuzot-Garcher C (2008) Changes in meibomian fatty acids and clinical signs in patients with meibomian gland dysfunction after minocycline treatment. Br J Ophthalmol 92(6):819–822

Stone DU, Chodosh J (2004) Oral tetracyclines for ocular rosacea: an evidence-based review of the literature. Cornea 23:106–109

Strong B, Farley W, Stern ME, Pflugfelder SC (2005) Topical cyclosporine inhibits conjunctival epithelial apoptosis in experimental murine keratoconjunctivitis sicca. Cornea 24(1):80–85

Ta CN, Shine WE, McCulley JP, Pandya A, Trattler W, Norbury JW (2003) Effects of minocycline on the ocular flora of patients with acne rosacea or seborrheic blepharitis. Cornea 22:545–548

Tamargo RJ, Bok RA, Brem H (1991) Angiogenesis inhibition by minocycline. Cancer Res 51:672–675

Torkildsen G (2009) The effects of lubricant eye drops on visual function as measured by the Inter-blink interval Visual Acuity Decay test. Clin Ophthalmol 3:501–506

Tsubota K, Goto E, Fujita H, Ono M, Inoue H, Saito I, Shimmura S (1999a) Treatment of dry eye by autologous serum application in Sjögren's syndrome. Br J Ophthalmol 83(4):390–395

Tsubota K, Goto E, Shimmura S et al (1999b) Treatment of persistent corneal epithelial defect by autologous serum application. Ophthalmology 106:1984–1989

Turner K, Pflugfelder SC, Ji Z, Fener WJ, Stern M, Reis BL (2000) Interleukin-6 levels in the conjunctival epithelium of patients with dry eye disease treated with cyclo- sporine ophthalmic emulsion. Cornea 19:492–496

Ubels JL, McCartney MD, Lantz WK, Beaird J, Dayalan A, Edelhauser HF (1995) Effects of preservative-free artificial tear solutions on corneal epithelial structure and function. Arch Ophthalmol 113(3):371–378

Veldman P, Colby K (2011) Current evidence for topical azithromycin 1% ophthalmic solution in the treatment of blepharitis and blepharitis-associated ocular dryness. Int Ophthalmol Clin 51(4):43–52

Yoo SE, Lee DC, Chang MH (2005) The effect of low-dose doxycycline therapy in chronic meibomian gland dysfunction. Korean J Ophthalmol 19:258–263

Yung YH, Toda I, Sakai C, Yoshida A, Tsubota K (2012) Punctal plugs for treatment of post-LASIK dry eye. Jpn J Ophthalmol 56(3):208–213

Zimmerman TJ, Kooner KS, Kandarakis AS, Ziegler SP (1984) Improving the therapeutic index of topically applied ocular drugs. Arch Ophthalmol 102(4):551–553

Surgical Management of Dry Eyes

6

Lingo Y. Lai, Clark L. Springs, and Richard A. Burgett

6.1 Tear Volume Underproduction

Tear volume underproduction can be secondary to:

- Systemic medication side effects
- Systemic autoimmune diseases affecting the lacrimal gland (e.g., Sjögren's syndrome)
- Iatrogenic lacrimal gland damage (e.g., post-radiation therapy for head and neck cancers)

The surgical interventions for eyes that have tear volume underproduction include methods that extend the amount of time tears remain on the ocular surface by blocking or narrowing the tear drainage system. However, if the lacrimal gland damage is very severe, lack of tear volume can result in severe ocular damage. In those cases, more advanced surgical options for managing severe ocular damage should be considered (see Sect. 6.4), such as lacrimal gland transplantation performed by an ophthalmic plastic surgical consultant.

Indications for utilizing these procedures to address tear volume underproduction include dry eyes that have mild to moderate improvement on artificial tears or if artificial tears are unable to be administered at the required frequency, either due to patient inability to administer eyedrops or due to schedule limitations. Patients who have intolerance to punctal plugs secondary to dysesthesia might also benefit from these surgical interventions.

6.1.1 Surgical Options

- Partial punctal occlusion with cautery

Pros

– *Decreases the size of punctum orifice* versus *creating a complete occlusion*

Cons

– *Nonreversible procedure*
– *Could result in epiphora*

Steps: Infratrochlear nerve block is first performed using 1 ml of 2 % lidocaine. The tip of the cautery device is inserted into the lacrimal punctum and transverses the horizontal portion of the lacrimal canaliculus. The device is engaged in close contact with the wall of the lacrimal punctum and canaliculus until a 0.5 mm or less orifice diameter of the lacrimal punctum remains. A few drops of normal saline are applied around the punctal tissue and the cautery tip if the tip remains

L.Y. Lai, MD (✉) • C.L. Springs, MD
Department of Ophthalmology, Glick Eye Institute,
Indiana University School of Medicine,
Indianapolis, IN, USA
e-mail: lingo.lai@yahoo.com; csprings@iupui.edu

R.A. Burgett, MD, FACS
Department of Ophthalmology, Indiana University
School of Medicine, Indianapolis, IN, USA
e-mail: rburgett@me.com

C. Chan (ed.), *Dry Eye: A Practical Approach*, Essentials in Ophthalmology,
DOI 10.1007/978-3-662-44106-0_6, © Springer-Verlag Berlin Heidelberg 2015

adherent to the tissue after thermocautery is complete. Prescribe antibiotic ointment to be used three times a day for 1 week (Holzchuh et al. 2011).

- Complete punctal occlusion with thermal cautery, diathermy, or laser coagulation

Pros

- *Larger effect than partial punctal occlusion, as punctum is completely occluded*

Cons

- *Nonreversible procedure*
- *Could result in epiphora*

Steps: Infratrochlear nerve block is first performed using 1 ml of 2 % lidocaine. The tip of the cautery device is inserted into the lacrimal punctum and transverses the horizontal portion of the lacrimal canaliculus. The device is engaged in close contact with the walls of the lacrimal punctum and canaliculus for 10–14 s. Satisfactory cautery is noted when the surrounding punctal tissue turns white. A few drops of normal saline are applied around the punctal tissue and the cautery tip if the tip remains adherent to the tissue after thermocautery is complete. Prescribe antibiotic ointment to be used three times a day for 1 week (Ohba et al. 2011).

> **Tip**
>
> Satisfactory cautery occurs when the surrounding punctal tissue turns white.

- Complete punctal occlusion with suturing

Pros

- *Theoretically higher success rate than punctal occlusion by cautery due to complete removal of punctal epithelium*

Cons

- *Nonreversible procedure*
- *Could result in epiphora*
- *Could have corneal irritation from suture*

Steps: Place 1 drop of topical anesthetic into the operative eye and inject 0.1 ml of 2 % Xylocaine with adrenaline into the tissues surrounding the punctum and the vertical portion of the canaliculus. Prepare and drape the surgical field in a sterile fashion. Use a corneal rust ring burr with a 0.6-mm diameter to remove the epithelium from the punctum and the vertical portion of the canaliculus to a depth of 2 mm. Complete removal of the punctal epithelium is essential. Place a simple interrupted 6-0 chromic suture using a 3/8 circle reverse-cutting needle to bring the raw surfaces together. Place this suture parallel to the lid margin to avoid corneal irritation. Schedule follow-up appointments at 1-, 3-, and 6-month intervals (Liu and Sadhan 2002).

> **Tip**
>
> Complete removal of the punctal epithelium is essential.

6.2 Tear Film Instability

Tear film instability causes increased evaporative losses and can be secondary to:

- Meibomian gland dysfunction
- Acute exacerbation of anterior or posterior blepharitis

Meibomian glands produce the lipid layer of the tear film, which overlies the aqueous portion of the tear film and prevents accelerated evaporation of tears. In eyes with severe anterior or posterior blepharitis, the meibomian glands become chronically plugged and are unable to effectively secrete the lipid layer, resulting in a deterioration of tear film quality. The surgical interventions for these eyes restore functionality of the meibomian glands.

Indications for surgical interventions to address tear film instability include moderate to severe meibomian gland dysfunction, which can manifest as decreased tear breakup time, meibomian gland plugging, lid margin telangiectasias, and hyperemia. These patients often complain of foreign body sensation and irritated eyes, with partial relief when using warm compresses. The surgical techniques described in this section utilize proprietary devices, which have accompanying published data in the literature to support their benefit in symptomatic patients.

6.2.1 Surgical Options

- Meibomian gland probing with Maskin probe

Pros
- *In-office procedure*
- *Repeatable procedure*

Cons
- *Severe cases of meibomian gland dysfunction may require multiple sessions.*
- *May have difficulty inserting Maskin probe into severely atrophied meibomian gland orifices.*

Studies: Maskin (2010) published a single center study ($n = 25$ patients) showing 96 % of patients had immediate post-probing relief and 100 % of patients had symptomatic relief by 4 weeks post-probing. Eighty percent of patients required only one treatment, and 20 % of patients required re-treatment at average of 4.6 months.

Steps: Evaluate patency of gland orifices, status of the glands (note signs of atrophy), length of the glands, and signs of ductal dilation with transillumination. Use either a 2- or 4-mm probe for the procedure. If the glands appear shorter in length, use the 2-mm probe. Place 1–2 drops of viscous topical anesthetic to the inferior conjunctival fornix, with sufficient anesthetic to cover the lid margin. Place a sterile cotton-tipped applicator soaked with 4 % lidocaine directly onto the lid margin throughout the procedure.

After adequate anesthesia is obtained, seat the patient at the slit lamp with an assistant supporting the patient's head against the forehead bar and allow the patient's chin to be in the chin rest in a comfortable position. Open the package containing the sterile probe and insert the probe handle into the hub of the probe cannula in order to remove the probe from the package. Place tension on the eyelid by using a finger or cotton-tipped applicator to gently pull the lid laterally and provide traction. With the opposite hand, hold the sterile probe handle like a pencil and rest the probe tip on the orifice. Advance the tip using short, fine, subtle "dart-throwing" movements in a perpendicular orientation to the lid margin. In cases of orifice metaplasia, a circular router movement can be used to find the orifice.

If the wire flexes during probing, the angle or placement within the orifice can be adjusted to allow penetration. If there is persistent tenderness or resistance after the 2-mm probe is used, perform transillumination again. If the length of the glands exceeds the length of the 4-mm probe, repeat the probing procedure using the 4-mm probe to relieve the resistance. Relief of intra-ductal resistance is associated with a perceptible "pop" and trickle of blood at the orifice. A plug of meibum can be noted to escape along the probe tip.

At the termination of the procedure, the probe should easily pass through the orifice and encounter no resistance along the way. A gritty sound and feel may occur during probing. Hemorrhage seen during probing can range from a dot to a fine trickle of blood at the lid margin. Patients with severe, chronic inflammation may have discomfort during the initial probing and could benefit from dividing the probing into multiple sessions, starting with probing of the 6–8 glands that have the most severe symptoms (Maskin 2010).

> **Tip**
>
> Prior to start of procedure, evaluate patency of gland orifices, status of the glands (note signs of atrophy), length of the glands, and signs of ductal dilation with transillumination.

- Meibomian gland probing with hyfrecator tip

Pros
- *In-office procedure*
- *Repeatable procedure*

Cons
- *Severe cases of meibomian gland dysfunction may require multiple sessions.*
- *May have difficulty inserting hyfrecator into severely atrophied meibomian gland orifices.*

Studies: Wladis (2012) published a single center study ($n = 10$ patients, 40 eyelids) showing 90 % of patients were able to successfully discontinue use of doxycycline at 1 month post-probing. OSDI (Ocular Surface Disease Index) questionnaire score showed statistically significant improvement at 1 month and 6 months post-procedure. No patients required re-treatment.

Steps: Inject all 4 eyelids using 2 % lidocaine with 1:100,000 epinephrine. Insert the hyfrecator tip into the meibomian gland orifice perpendicular to the eyelid margin. Advance the probe until a faint "pop" is felt, which indicates release of the cicatrized orifice. Continue advancing the probe and look for egress of normal meibomian gland contents. On termination of the procedure, faint petechial hemorrhages should be visible at the meibomian gland orifices (Wladis 2012).

> **Tip**
>
> A faint "pop" can be felt, indicating release of the cicatrized meibomian gland orifice.

- LipiFlow system

Pros
- *In-office procedure*
- *Repeatable procedure*
- *Does not require probing meibomian gland orifices with any device (theoretically improved patient comfort)*

Cons
- *Severe cases of meibomian gland dysfunction may require multiple sessions.*
- *Cost.*

Studies: Greiner (2012) published a single center study ($n = 21$ patients, 42 eyes) that showed statistically significant improvement in OSDI questionnaire score, SPEED (Standard Patient Evaluation for Eye Dryness) questionnaire score, meibomian gland secretion score, and tear breakup time at 1 month, with improvement maintained at 9 months post-procedure. All patients received single 12-min LipiFlow treatment in each eye.

Lane et al. (2012) published a multicenter clinical trial comparing safety and effectiveness of LipiFlow versus iHeat Warm Compress for adults with meibomian gland dysfunction ($n = 69$ LipiFlow, 90 iHeat Warm Compress). The LipiFlow group showed a statistically significant improvement in meibomian gland secretion, as well as in tear breakup time, at 2 and 4 weeks.

Steps: The LipiFlow system has two parts: the Disposable (ocular component) and the Handheld Control System. The Disposable has two parts: a lid warmer and an eyecup. Anesthetize the eye with topical proparacaine eyedrops. Insert the Disposable in a similar fashion to insertion of a sclera lens or surgical corneal protector. Instruct the patient to keep the eyes closed prior to initiating treatment in order to ensure correct device position on the eyelids. At initiation of the treatment, the inflatable air bladder of the eyecup will inflate, compressing the eyelids between the heated lid warmer and the air bladder. During the treatment, the air bladder will inflate and deflate, massaging the eyelids from the terminal end of the meibomian glands toward the direction of the meibomian gland orifice. Continue treatment for 12 min (Greiner 2012; Lane et al. 2012).

6.3 Mechanical Disturbance

Mechanical disturbances are varied and mainly involve the conjunctiva or the eyelid. Mechanical disturbances cause increased evaporative loss, abnormal drainage of tears, or prolonged corneal exposure time and can be secondary to:
- Conjunctivochalasis
- Lower eyelid malpositions (e.g., ectropion, entropion)
- Eyelid dysfunctions (e.g., lagophthalmos, exposure keratopathy)

Conjunctivochalasis is characterized by the presence of excessive folds of conjunctiva and is frequently associated with dry eye, although the exact relationship remains unknown. It usually involves the lower bulbar conjunctiva, though the superior bulbar conjunctiva can be affected as well. Severity of conjunctivochalasis is correlated with severity of symptoms. Mild to moderate conjunctivochalasis can mimic dry eye due to tear film disruption and instability. In severe conjunctivochalasis, the redundant conjunctiva physically obstructs the lower punctum and interferes with lid blinking and closure, causing symptoms of epiphora. Surgical removal or repositioning of

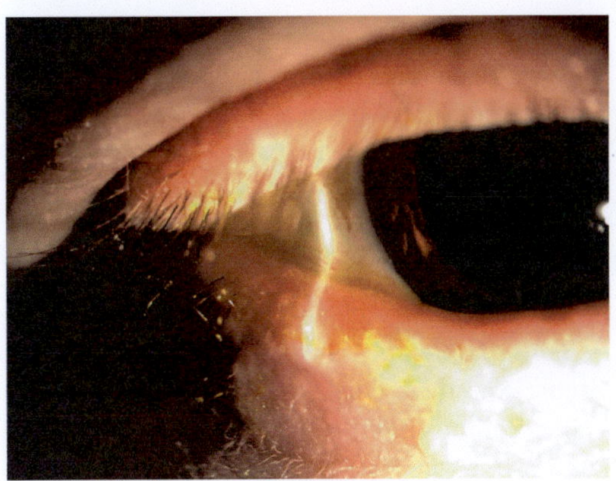

Fig. 6.1 Inferior conjunctivochalasis

the excessive conjunctiva eliminates the mechanical disturbance (Fig. 6.1).

The primary indication for surgical intervention for conjunctivochalasis is intolerance of foreign body sensation. The most common locations of excess conjunctiva causing symptoms include inferiorly and inferotemporally. Patients often report foreign body sensation or localized epiphora sensation in that region of their eyes. The following section describes various techniques to remove the excess conjunctiva. Although some studies have been published comparing techniques, there is no strong evidence in the literature that one surgical technique is substantially better than the other. Most surgeons choose one or two techniques based on their comfort level and make modifications based on their individual post-op results.

6.3.1 Surgical Options

- Conjunctivochalasis resection

Pros
- *Reapproximates normal conjunctival anatomy*

Cons
- *Requires suture placement*

Steps: Anesthetize the eye with topical proparacaine eyedrops. Prep and drape the eye and insert a lid speculum. Inject 1 % lidocaine in the inferior subconjunctival region. Make an arc-like incision in the inferior bulbar conjunctiva approximately 2 mm from the corneal limbus. Excise the subconjunctival tissues distally from the arc-like incision to the extent of the redundant conjunctiva. Make radial incisions to divide the conjunctiva into nasal, central, and temporal blocks. Resect the redundant conjunctiva in each block based on the extent of redundancy. Close the central block first, using 8-0 Vicryl interrupted sutures. The remaining two blocks should be sutured closed with adjustments to maintain appropriate shape and tension for smooth junctions between the blocks and to obtain a good tear meniscus. Prescribe topical 0.5 % levofloxacin and 0.1 % fluorometholone eyedrops for 1 month. Remove stitches at 1 week postoperatively (Hara et al. 2011).

- Conjunctivochalasis resection with cautery

Pros
- *Better adherence of conjunctiva because of cautery*

Cons
- *Theoretically increased scarring because of cautery*
- *Removal of nylon suture required*

Steps: Anesthetize the eye with topical proparacaine eyedrops and subconjunctival 2 % lidocaine. Use ophthalmic microscissors to make a semicircular incision from 3 o'clock to 9 o'clock position in the inferior conjunctiva approximately 0.5 mm from the corneal limbus. Leave angle of 45° at the two ends of the incision. Use an iris repository and microforceps to push the loose conjunctiva from the inferior fornix onto the corneal surface. The redundant conjunctiva will be seen overlapping onto the inferior corneal surface. Make a second curved incision into the redundant conjunctiva and parallel to the first incision. This creates a semiperitomy strip of redundant conjunctiva that should be excised in close proximity to the 0.5-mm conjunctiva flap adjacent to the inferior corneal limbus. Place gentle cautery in two lines (12–18 spots in zigzag pattern) subconjunctivally under the incision to form tight adhesions with the underlying sclera along the corneal limbus. Use 10-0 nylon suture to close the incision at 3 o'clock and 9 o'clock positions. Remove the sutures at 1 week postoperatively (Wang et al. 2012).

- Conjunctival resection with paste-pinch-cut technique

Pros
- *Possible decrease in intraoperative time because it does not require suturing*
- *Similar technique to modern pterygium excision with autograft*

Cons
- *Risk of glued wound becoming unsealed*

Steps: Anesthetize the eye with topical proparacaine eyedrops. Prep and drape the eye and insert a lid speculum. Inject 2 % lidocaine with epinephrine in the inferior subconjunctival region. Use a methylene blue pen to place an arc-like marking approximately 5–6 mm inferior to the limbus. Use Westcott scissors to make a small buttonhole in the temporal bulbar conjunctiva at the edge of the pen marking. Use a 19-gauge cannula to inject 0.3 ml of the fibrinogen component of fibrin sealant (Tisseel; Baxter AG Industries, Vienna, Austria) through the buttonhole subconjunctivally along the pen marking. Inject 0.3 ml of the thrombin component in a similar fashion. Immediately after injection of the thrombin sealant, use modified (curved) ptosis forceps to pinch the conjunctiva and hold for 20 s. This step gathers the excess conjunctiva and subconjunctiva sealant into a ridge and allows the sealant to polymerize. After 20 s, use Westcott scissors to excise the ridge, leaving a sealed wound 2–3 mm inferior to the limbus. Prescribe antibiotic eyedrops to use three times a day for 1 week and steroid eyedrops to use three times a day for 3 weeks. Schedule follow-up appointments at 1-day, 1-month, and 3-month intervals (Doss et al. 2012).

> **Tip**
>
> Immediately after injection of the thrombin sealant, use modified (curved) ptosis forceps to pinch the conjunctiva and hold for 20 s. This step gathers the excess conjunctiva and subconjunctiva sealant into a ridge and allows the sealant to polymerize.

- Conjunctival resection with sutured amniotic membrane transplantation

Pros
- *Reapproximates normal conjunctival anatomy*

Cons
- *Requires suture placement*
- *Cost of amniotic membrane graft*

Steps: Anesthetize the eye with topical proparacaine eyedrops. Prep and drape the eye and insert a lid speculum. Inject 2 % lidocaine with epinephrine in the inferior subconjunctival region. Make a peritomy of the inferior conjunctiva 1 mm from the limbus. Use Westcott scissors to excise the loose and redundant conjunctiva. Place amniotic membrane transplant over the conjunctival defect and trim off excess membrane. Place a continuous suture using 10-0 nylon to approximate the conjunctival edges with the amniotic membrane. Place a mixed antibiotic steroid ointment into the operative eye and then patch the eye. Remove the eye patch on postoperative day one. Prescribe artificial tears, steroid, and antibiotic eyedrops to use five times a day until full epithelialization of the amniotic membrane, which usually occurs in 2 weeks. Remove the suture at 2 weeks postoperatively. Discontinue steroid and antibiotic eyedrops 3–4 days after suture removal. Continue artificial tears for at least 1 month (Georgiadis and Terzidou 2001).

- Conjunctival resection with fibrin glue amniotic membrane transplantation

Pros
- *Possible decrease in intraoperative time because it does not require suturing*
- *Similar technique to modern pterygium excision with allograft*

Cons
- *Risk of glued wound becoming unsealed*

Steps: Anesthetize the eye with topical 2 % lidocaine gel and a few drops of non-preserved 1:1,000 epinephrine for hemostasis. Prep and drape the eye and insert a lid speculum. Make an arc-like inferior conjunctival peritomy 1–2 mm posterior to the limbus. Place traction suture using a 7-0 Vicryl placed 2 mm posterior to the limbus at 6 o'clock position and rotate the eye upward. Look for loose conjunctiva that is easily mobile using forceps. Trim off areas of severely thinned conjunctiva. Apply the amniotic membrane over the conjunctival defect, with the membrane stromal side toward the sclera. Fold back half of the amniotic membrane. Apply thrombin solution to the sclera surface, and apply fibrinogen solution to the stromal surface of the membrane. Flip the membrane back onto the sclera and use a muscle hook over the membrane to spread the fibrin glue that is under the membrane. Repeat the above steps for the other half of the amniotic membrane. Trim the excess amniotic membrane and fibrin so that the membrane is flush with the conjunctiva (Kheirkhah et al. 2007).

> **Tip**
> Apply thrombin solution to the sclera surface and apply fibrinogen solution to the stromal surface of the membrane. Flip the membrane back onto the scleral and use a muscle hook over the membrane to spread the fibrin glue that is under the membrane.

- No conjunctival resection/suture-only technique

Pros
- *No conjunctival excision required*

Cons
- *Risk of globe perforation when suturing excess conjunctiva to sclera*

Steps: Anesthetize the eye with topical proparacaine eyedrops. Prep and drape the eye and insert a lid speculum. Inject 2 % lidocaine with epinephrine in the inferior subconjunctival region. Place three interrupted 6-0 Vicryl sutures 8 mm posterior from the limbus, attaching the bulbar conjunctiva to the sclera. Take care not to perforate the globe. The normal anatomic depth of the inferior fornix is 8 mm from the limbus. Avoid going farther than 8 mm, as restriction of lower gaze may occur. Vicryl suture is ideal for this procedure because it permits focal inflammation to occur so that the forniceal conjunctiva

will firmly attach to the globe (Otaka and Kyu 2000).

> **Tip**
> The normal anatomic depth of the inferior fornix is 8 mm from the limbus. Avoid going farther than 8 mm, as restriction of lower gaze may occur.

Lower eyelid malpositions, such as ectropion and entropion, can create either a dry eye syndrome or symptomatic epiphora. Corneal exposure from ectropion or irritation from lashes touching the cornea in entropion creates corneal irritation with a constellation of dry eye symptoms. Epiphora can result from reflex hypersecretion but can also occur from lacrimal pump failure or the inability of tears to enter a malpositioned or stenotic punctum. Lower eyelid malposition, whether ectropion or entropion, is commonly caused by involutional changes most commonly related to aging. Repair of these malpositions involves tightening the horizontal eyelid supports, namely, the tarsus and lateral canthal tendon. Repair of a dehiscent lower eyelid retractor band can restore vertical support in the eyelid and restore the tarsus to a favorable anatomic position. Techniques for managing involutional lower eyelid malpositions are summarized below and may be addressed by the general ophthalmic surgeon.

Floppy eyelid syndrome represents a pathologic end spectrum of involutional eyelid disease and may require special techniques and experience. Eyelid malpositions related to scarring (cicatricial disease) should be surgically managed in a significantly different manner. Skin disorders that result in skin tightening (i.e., scleroderma, burns, radiation) frequently cause ectropion, while conjunctival scarring diseases (i.e., Stevens-Johnson syndrome, trachoma, ocular cicatricial pemphigoid) cause entropion or trichiasis. In many cases, the management of cicatricial malpositions requires the addition of the deficient eyelid lamella, namely, skin for ectropion and mucous membrane for entropion, which are beyond the scope of this manual. Cicatricial changes from overcorrected ptosis repair or lower eyelid blepharoplasty may have scarring in more than one lamella and can be challenging. The approach of these cicatricial malpositions is not described below, and these patients warrant a referral to an ophthalmic plastic surgeon.

Indications for surgical intervention in lower eyelid malpositions include horizontal lower eyelid laxity, corneal decompensation from eyelashes rubbing against corneal surface, or persistent epiphora. Although some studies have been published comparing techniques, there is no strong evidence in the literature that one surgical technique is substantially better than the other. Most surgeons choose a technique based on their comfort level and make modifications based on their individual post-op results.

6.3.2 Surgical Options

- Ectropion repair via formal lateral tarsal strip procedure

Pros
- *Good visualization of tarsus to attach to periosteum for better reapproximation and creation of new lateral canthal angle*

Cons
- *More time intensive*

Steps: Inject 2 % lidocaine with 1:100,000 epinephrine to the lower eyelid. Prep and drape the eye. Instill tetracaine and place a corneal protector. Make a 1-cm lateral canthotomy incision using a No. 15 Bard-Parker blade. Use straight scissors to perform an inferior cantholysis. Pull the lower eyelid laterally and use a marking pen to indicate the target amount of horizontal shortening. Resect the epithelium overlying the lid margin of the planned tarsal strip. Use scissors to divide the eyelid into two lamellae at the gray line. Remove the skin of the anterior lamella to expose the tarsus. Cut the conjunctiva along the inferior edge of the tarsus to create a strip of tarsus. Remove the conjunctiva from the newly created tarsal strip with scalpel or Beaver blade. Place a suture using 5-0 Vicryl or 4-0 Prolene to attach the tarsal strip to the internal lateral orbital periosteum at a slight angle so that it is a little

higher compared to the height of the corresponding medial canthus. Approximate the upper and lower eyelid margins laterally using interrupted sutures. Close the canthotomy incision with absorbable sutures. Remove the corneal protector, either at completion of the procedure or prior to tying the canthal suspension suture. Apply ophthalmic antibiotic ointment to the incision site for 1–2 weeks (Anderson and Gordy 1979; Tse and Negg 2001).

- Ectropion repair via lateral wedge excision (Figs. 6.2, 6.3, 6.4, and 6.5)

Pros
- *Quick procedure*

Cons
- *Need to orient scissors in correct angle when making full-thickness block excision of eyelid to ensure better cosmetic result when reforming lateral canthal angle*

Steps: Inject 2 % lidocaine with 1:100,000 epinephrine to the lower eyelid. Prep and drape the eye. Instill tetracaine and a corneal protector. Make a 1-cm lateral canthotomy incision using a No. 15 Bard-Parker blade. Use straight scissors to perform an inferior cantholysis. Retract the eyelid laterally to estimate the horizontal redundancy in the lid with care to avoid excessive lengthening of the medial canthal tendon. Use straight scissors for a full-thickness block excision of the redundant excessive eyelid. Achieve hemostasis with cautery. Engage the cut tarsal edge with a 5-0 Prolene or 5-0 Vicryl. With retraction of the upper limb of the canthal tendon and protection of the orbital tissue with cotton-tipped applicator or small malleable retractor, pass the Prolene suture in a medial to lateral direction to engage the internal orbital rim periosteum. A sharp canthal angle can be reformed by adding a chromic suture which brings the two gray lines into apposition in the open canthotomy wound prior to tying the Prolene canthal suspension suture. Close the canthotomy incision with absorbable sutures. Remove the corneal protector, either at the end of the procedure or prior to tying the canthal suspension suture. Apply ophthalmic antibiotic ointment to the incision site for 1–2 weeks (Tse and Negg 2001).

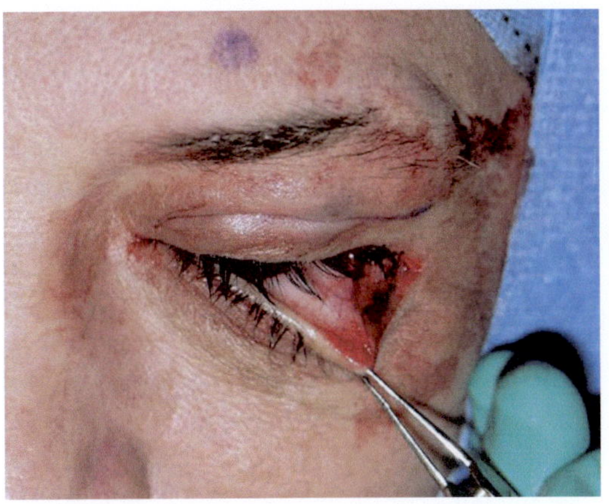

Fig. 6.2 A lateral canthotomy and inferior cantholysis have been made

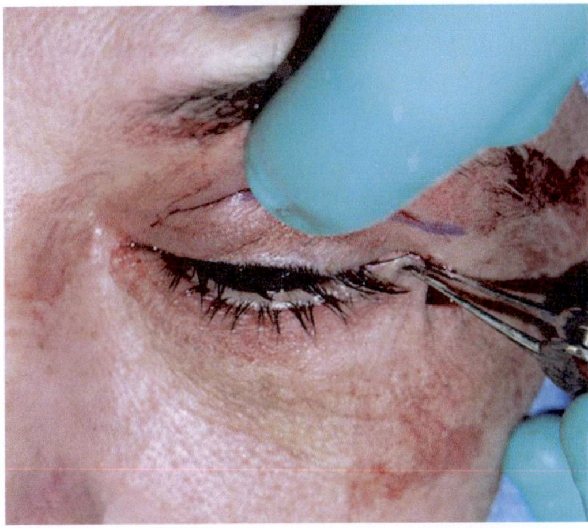

Fig. 6.3 Retract the eyelid laterally to estimate the horizontal redundancy in the eyelid

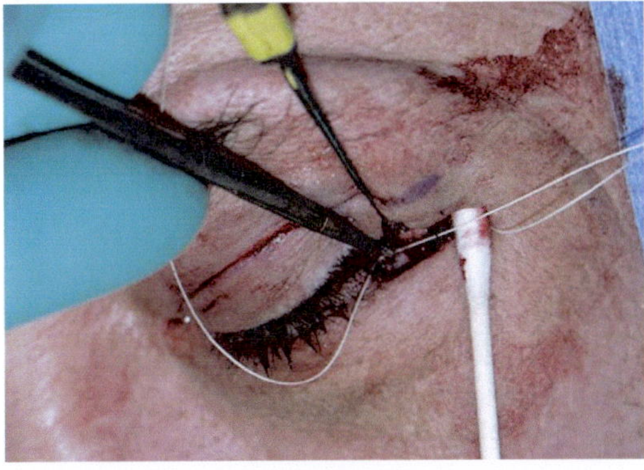

Fig. 6.4 Pass the Prolene suture in a medial to lateral direction to engage the internal orbital rim periosteum. Use a cotton-tipped applicator to protect the orbital tissue and a retractor to gently lift upward the upper limb of the canthal tendon for better exposure

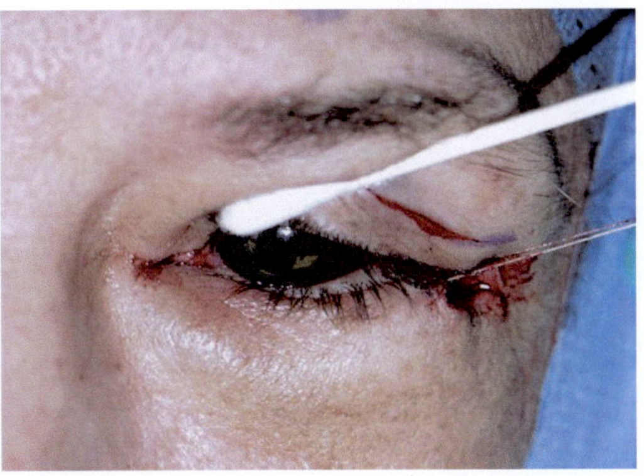

Fig. 6.5 The canthal angle should be sharp, with the two gray lines in apposition

> **Tip**
> Orient scissors in correct angle when making full-thickness block excision of the redundant excessive eyelid to ensure better cosmetic result of new lateral canthal angle.

- Entropion repair, anterior approach

Pros
- *Quick procedure*

Cons
- *Skin incision gives potential for visible scar and scleral show.*

Steps: Inject 2 % lidocaine with 1:100,000 epinephrine to the lower eyelid. Prep and drape the eye. Instill tetracaine and place the corneal protector. Make a subciliary incision 2–3 mm below the eyelash line from a point inferior to the punctum to the lateral canthus and connect it to a canthotomy incision. Separate a skin-muscle flap away from the posterior lamella. Perform a horizontal tightening procedure as indicated above. Verify hemostasis. If dehiscence of the retractor band is noted, repair of the retractors to the inferior border of tarsus may be indicated. Redrape the skin-muscle flap of the lower eyelid and excise the excess. Close the subciliary-canthotomy incision with absorbable suture. Remove the corneal protector, either at the end of the procedure or prior to tying the canthal suspension suture. Apply ophthalmic antibiotic ointment to the incision site. Remove the sutures at 1 week postoperatively (Kronish 2001).

• Entropion repair, posterior approach

Pros

– *Horizontal incision is done transconjunctivally.*

Cons

– *More time intensive*

Steps: Inject 2 % lidocaine with 1:100,000 epinephrine to the lower eyelid. Prep and drape the eye. Instill tetracaine and a corneal protector. Perform canthotomy incision, cantholysis, and resection/preparation for horizontal tightening as indicated above. Visualize the posterior lamella with retraction. Look for the common dehiscence of the retractor band. Use Westcott scissors first as a blunt dissector and then as scissors to make a horizontal conjunctival incision. If conjunctiva is excessive, a thin strip may be trimmed to the inferior pole of tarsus. Reattach the retractor band to the inferior pole of tarsus to bring the tarsus back into proper vertical orientation with 6-0 Vicryl sutures on a spatulated needle. Resuspend the eyelid via a horizontal tightening procedure of choice as above. Close the canthotomy incision with absorbable sutures. Remove the corneal protector, either at the end of the case or prior to tying the canthal suspension suture. Apply ophthalmic antibiotic ointment to the incision site for 1–2 weeks (Dresner and Karesh 1993; Kronish 2001; Tse and Negg 2001).

> **Tip**
> Visualize the posterior lamella with retraction and look for the common dehiscence of the retractor band.

Eyelid dysfunctions can occur secondary to facial nerve palsies, in which there is incomplete lid closure or incomplete blink. Lagophthalmos can also be seen secondary to severe proptosis in thyroid-related eye disease. Both scenarios result in exposure keratopathy and dry eye symptoms.

Indications for tarsorrhaphy in eyelid dysfunctions include persistent dry eye symptoms, corneal decompensation (often manifesting as neurotrophic

ulcer), or patient inability to administer artificial tears at required frequent dosing. Temporary tarsorrhaphy should be utilized in cases where the eyelid dysfunction is expected to improve in weeks, such as with post-op neurotrophic ulcers or exposure keratopathy in intubated intensive care unit patients. Permanent tarsorrhaphy is the best approach in patients who need the tarsorrhaphy in place for months to years. For both types of tarsorrhaphies, studies have been published comparing various techniques. However, there is no strong evidence in the literature that one surgical technique is better than the other. Most surgeons choose a technique on par with their comfort level and make modifications based on their individual post-op results. One useful surgical technique for temporary tarsorrhaphy is detailed here. One surgical technique for permanent tarsorrhaphy that is commonly used by ophthalmic plastic surgeons is detailed below.

6.3.3 Surgical Options

• Temporary tarsorrhaphy with bolsters (drawstring technique) or without bolsters

Pros

– *Easily reversible*
– *Can be performed at bedside or in the clinic*
– *With drawstring technique, can easily loosen or tighten as needed to visualize the cornea*

Cons

– *Potential risk of infection from suture; suture may need to be replaced every 2–3 weeks.*
– *Not cosmetically ideal (very visible suture).*

Steps: Inject 2 % lidocaine with 1:100,000 epinephrine to the upper and lower eyelids. Prep and drape the eye. Instill tetracaine and a corneal protector. Create sterile bolster material by cutting a Foley catheter into 2 semicircular strips. One of the strips is then cut into two 2-cm sections and one 1-cm section. The 2-cm sections are the bolsters for the upper and lower eyelids. The 1-cm section allows for closure of the drawstring when placed against the bolster of the lower eyelid. Place a double-armed 6-0

Prolene on a P-3 cutting needle through one of the 2-cm bolsters at 2 mm from the end. Place the needle 3–4 mm from the upper eyelid margin into the tarsus and exiting the eyelid margin at the gray line. Place the needle into the gray line of the lower eyelid margin and exit the lower eyelid 2–3 mm inferior to the eyelid margin. Using the other end of the double-armed 6-0 Prolene suture, choose a location lateral from the initial needle pass and place the needle 3–4 mm from the upper eyelid margin into the tarsus, exiting the eyelid margin at the gray line. Then place the needle into the gray line of the lower eyelid margin immediately inferior to the upper eyelid lateral needle pass location and exit the lower eyelid 2–3 mm inferior to the eyelid margin. Pass both ends of the double-armed 6-0 Prolene through the second 2-cm bolster (for the lower eyelid). Pass both ends of the double-armed 6-0 Prolene through the 1-cm bolster. Remove the needles and tie the two ends of the suture, leaving 2–3 cm of slack in the suture. To perform temporary tarsorrhaphy without bolsters, follow the above steps but without incorporating bolsters in each step (Kitchens et al. 2002).

- Permanent lateral tarsorrhaphy via intermarginal adhesion technique

Pros
– *Cosmetically acceptable*

Cons
– *More time intensive and should be performed in the operating room.*
– *Procedure can be reversed, but reversal should be performed in the operating room.*

Steps: Inject 2 % lidocaine with 1:100,000 epinephrine to the upper and lower eyelids. Prep and drape the eye. Instill tetracaine and a corneal protector. Use a #64 Beaver blade to make two incisions at the eyelid margin through skin but not tarsus in both upper and lower eyelids. The lateral incisions should be at the lateral canthus. The medial incisions should be placed at a position commensurate with the desired position and aggressiveness of the desired tarsorrhaphy. Use a sharp Westcott scissors (or blade) to resect the epithelium at the lateral eyelid margins between the two vertical incisions. Pass a 5-0 or 6-0 Vicryl in a horizontal mattress fashion

with the knot oriented toward the lateral canthus to bring the tarsal plates into apposition. Place a second suture if required. Assure that no suture material is exposed from the posterior lamella. Remove the corneal protector. Tie the tarsorrhaphy suture(s). The same suture can then be passed in a horizontal mattress fashion with an externalized knot to support the internally placed suture with entry and exit points in the lash line and with tarsal engagement with the suture pass. Apply ophthalmic antibiotic ointment to the incision site for 1–2 weeks.

> **Tip**
> Pass the suture in a horizontal mattress fashion with the knot oriented toward the lateral canthus to bring the tarsal plates into apposition. Place a second suture if required. Assure that no suture material is exposed from the posterior lamella.

6.4 Ocular Surface Damage

Ocular surface damage can be secondary to:
- Systemic autoimmune diseases affecting the mucous membranes (e.g., ocular cicatricial pemphigoid)
- Limbal cell deficiency from severe ocular burns
- Limbal cell deficiency from Stevens-Johnson syndrome (SJS) and toxic epidermal necrolysis (TEN)
- Graft-versus-host disease after bone marrow transplantation

In most cases of ocular surface damage that require advanced surgical interventions, the cornea cannot repair itself due to destruction of the limbal cell population. Surgical techniques for ocular surface reconstruction include conjunctival limbal autograft (CLAU), living-related conjunctival limbal allograft (lr-CLAL), keratolimbal allograft (KLAL), and combined conjunctival limbal and keratolimbal allograft (C-KLAL). CLAU is a surgical procedure that transplants limbal tissue attached to a conjunctival carrier from the healthy eye of the patient to the contralateral stem-cell-deficient eye. Since this is an autograft procedure, systemic immunosuppression is not required postoperatively. This procedure is a good choice for unilateral limbal cell deficiency. Since CLAU is an autograft procedure that does not require systemic immunosuppression postoperatively, it is an appropriate surgical intervention a general ophthalmic surgeon can provide. In addition, for acute cases of ocular surface damage secondary to Stevens-Johnson, toxic epidermal necrolysis, or severe ocular burns, immediate surgical intervention using amniotic membrane grafts can drastically improve the patient's visual prognosis, and this surgical technique can be easily performed by a general ophthalmic surgeon. In non-acute scenarios, all forms of ocular surface inflammation must be well controlled for at least 6 months prior to surgical intervention.

Living-related conjunctival limbal allograft involves transplanting normal limbal tissue on a conjunctival carrier harvested from a living relative of the patient to the patient's diseased eye. KLAL is a surgical procedure that involves limbal tissue attached to a cornea carrier harvested from two cadaveric eyes and transplanted to the patient's diseased eye. C-KLAL is a combined procedure that transplants both limbal tissues attached to a cornea carrier harvested from a cadaveric eye, as well as conjunctival limbal autografts from a living relative of the patient. C-KLAL, KLAL, and lr-CLAL all require lifelong systemic immunosuppression postoperatively, as these are allograft transplants. Such patients often require interdisciplinary coordination of care with other specialties for postoperative management. These advanced surgical techniques are listed below to provide the general ophthalmic surgeon with understanding of the management for these patients but are best left to ophthalmic cornea surgeons comfortable with managing limbal cell transplants.

In cases of severe ocular damage, a substantial amount of forniceal scarring can occur. Some of the surgeries involving forniceal reconstruction are best performed by an ophthalmic plastic surgeon and are briefly mentioned here without detailed surgical steps.

6.4.1 Surgical Options

- Amniotic membrane grafting with fibrin glue

Pros
- *Similar technique to modern pterygium excision with allograft*

Cons
- *Cost*

Steps: Anesthetize the eye with topical proparacaine eyedrops. Prep and drape the eye and insert a lid speculum. Inject 2 % lidocaine with epinephrine in the inferior subconjunctival region. Dissect away adhesions to expose bare sclera. Remove subconjunctival fibrovascular tissue without excision of conjunctival tissue. Excise any scar tissue around the insertion of the rectus muscles to allow a freely mobile globe. Use cautery to achieve hemostasis of the sclera bed. Approximate the graft area and trim the amniotic membrane to a size slightly larger than the graft area size. Note and include areas in the fornices that may need amniotic membrane grafting as well. A Desmarres retractor may be needed to allow greater access to the superior fornix. Place the amniotic membrane stromal side up onto the cornea. Apply thrombin solution to the sclera surface and apply fibrinogen solution to the stromal surface of the amniotic membrane. Use forceps to flip the amniotic membrane back onto the sclera and use a muscle hook to spread the fibrin glue under the membrane. Use the muscle hook to push the amniotic membrane graft deep into the fornix to create an anatomically deep fornix. If forniceal placement of amniotic membrane is needed, place those membranes first, with the membrane stromal side against the tarsus. Continue topical antibiotic and steroid eyedrops postoperatively (Muqit et al. 2007).

- Amniotic membrane grafting with suture

Pros

– *Graft will not be dislodged with suture in place.*

Cons

– *More time intensive*

Steps: Anesthetize the eye with topical proparacaine eyedrops. Prep and drape the eye and insert a lid speculum. Inject 2 % lidocaine with epinephrine in the inferior subconjunctival region. Place the amniotic membrane stromal side up onto the cornea. Use the muscle hook to push the amniotic membrane graft deep into the fornix to create an anatomically deep fornix. Place mattress sutures using three double-ended 6-0 Dexon or Vicryl to secure the amniotic membrane graft to the upper eyelid margin. Use a Desmarres retractor to double-evert the upper eyelid and place superior fornix bolster sutures below the upper brow using 3-0 Prolene. The needle should pass from the amniotic membrane surface through the superior fornix and then through the full thickness of the upper eyelid. A gray line traction suture can also be placed to assist in everting the upper eyelid. Spread the free border of the amniotic membrane across the ocular surface. Repeat the previous steps to anchor the amniotic membrane and cover the inferior fornix and inferior tarsus. Continue topical antibiotic and steroid eyedrops postoperatively (Muqit et al. 2007).

> **Tip**
>
> Use Desmarres retractor to double-evert the upper eyelid and place superior fornix bolster sutures below the upper brow. The needle should pass from the amniotic membrane surface through the superior fornix and then through the full thickness of the upper eyelid.

• Conjunctival flap (total, pedicle, advancement)

Pros

– *Inexpensive (no cost of allograft)*

Cons

– *Cosmetically displeasing*

Steps: Evaluate conjunctival mobility preoperatively in the clinic. Anesthetize the eye with retrobulbar anesthesia. Prep and drape the eye and insert a lid speculum. Remove corneal epithelium using gentle mechanical debridement with surgical blade or dry cellulose sponge. Place a 4-0 or 6-0 silk limbal traction suture at 12 o'clock position to infraduct the eye. Use Westcott scissors or surgical blade to perform a complete peritomy. Use calipers to measure at least 14 mm from superior limbus into fornix to delineate the area necessary to completely cover the cornea. Inject 2 % lidocaine with 1:100,000 epinephrine into the subconjunctival space to mechanically separate the conjunctiva from the underlying Tenon's capsule. Infraduct the eye and make a 2-cm-long incision in the superior fornix 14 mm from and concentric to the limbus. Dissect conjunctiva to remove Tenon's capsule completely. Remove the superior limbal suture. Mobilize the flap onto the debrided corneal surface. Make relaxing incisions at the 4 o'clock and 8 o'clock positions to bring the flap into position without tension. Place interrupted sutures using Vicryl or nylon to secure the flap which completely covers the corneal surface. Bipedicle, single pedicle, and advancement flaps are created in similar steps (Vieira and Mannis 2011).

• Conjunctival grafting from oral mucosa (buccal, labial, hard palate)

Steps: Using buccal mucosa: Harvest a 15-mm (length) by 5-mm (height) piece of buccal mucosa from the upper gingivobuccal sulcus, as the glands in those areas have higher flow rates than those in other intraoral regions. Suture the harvested mucosa to the inferior fornix conjunctiva (Güerrissi and Belmonte 2004).

• Conjunctival grafting from nasal mucosa (septal, turbinate) or paranasal mucosa (maxillary sinus)

Steps: Using nasal mucosa: Performed under general anesthesia. Pack the nasal cavity for 5 min with gauze soaked in 2 % lidocaine with epinephrine (1:10,000 dilution) to anesthetize and decongest the nasal mucosa. Disinfect the midface and nasal cavity, and then inject 0.4 ml of local anesthetic into the submucosa of the inferior or middle turbinate harvest site. After 5 min, use a surgical blade to incise either the free edge of the inferior turbinate or the posterior third of the middle turbinate. Use a curved scissor to elevate and dissect off the mucosa. A bipolar cautery can be used for bleeding control. Pack the nasal cavity with Merocell or similar packing material for 48 h to stop the bleeding and stabilize the turbinate. After removal of the nasal pack, nasal dressing should be applied every 3 days for a length of 2 weeks to control crust formation at the harvest site. No oral or intranasal medication is needed.

Use straight scissors to strip off adjacent bone remnants and cavernous tissue from the excised nasal mucosa tissue. Trim the full-thickness nasal mucosa into thin and flat split-thickness grafts 1–2 mm in thickness. Wash the harvested grafts with normal saline and wrap them in wet gauze prior to autotransplant.

Perform a peritomy of the conjunctiva near the perilimbal region. If symblepharon is present, dissect and free away Tenon's capsule from the symblepharon. Apply mitomycin C 0.04 % soaked in microsponges for 4 min inside the deep fornix, avoiding bare sclera. Irrigate thoroughly with normal saline. Cover the large areas of bare bulbar sclera with amniotic membrane transplants (stromal side down), with fibrin sealants. Place the split-thickness autologous nasal mucosa epithelial side up on the perilimbal areas of the bulbar conjunctiva. Secure the nasal mucosa autotransplants with 10-0 nylon interrupted sutures. Four anchoring sutures in the upper and lower eyelids can be placed to prevent the collapse and contraction of recessed conjunctival tissues (Chun et al. 2011).

- Autologous oral mucosal epithelial transplantation

Steps: Obtain autologous oral mucosal epithelial cells from a 6-mm-diameter biopsy specimen from the patient's buccal mucosa. Culture the cells on an amniotic membrane spread on the bottom of a culture insert and coculture with mitomycin-C-inactivated 3T3 fibroblasts. Submerge the cultured cells in medium for approximately 1 week and then lower the medium level for 1–2 days. Expose an area of bare sclera and transplant the amniotic membrane to the area. Give systemic corticosteroids and cyclosporine to prevent postoperative inflammation and immunological response and taper dosing based on clinical findings. Prescribe steroid and antibiotic eyedrops to be used four times a day. A therapeutic soft contact lens can be used for at least 1 month to protect transplanted epithelium from mechanical ablation (Sotozono et al. 2013).

- Salivary gland transplantation

Steps: It is best to perform this procedure in a two-team approach to minimize ischemic time of the transplant. Harvest the submandibular gland with its supplying blood vessels and excretory duct, using a combined cervical and intraoral approach in the donor. Create a pocket in the temporal muscle of the recipient. Identify and dissect the superficial temporal vein and artery. Transfer the gland and anastomize the blood vessels microsurgically. Lead the excretory duct subcutaneously to the lateral canthus and implant it to the lateral fornix of the conjunctiva (Jacobsen et al. 2013).

- Limbal stem cell transplantation via conjunctival limbal autograft (CLAU)

Pros
- *Similar technique to modern pterygium excision with autograft*

Cons
- *Risk of limbal stem deficiency in donor eye*

Steps: Anesthetize both the recipient and donor eyes with topical proparacaine eyedrops. Prep and drape both eyes. Place a lid speculum in the recipient eye. Inject 2 % lidocaine with epinephrine in the subconjunctival region. Perform a conjunctival peritomy. Undermine the conjunctiva so it can recess posteriorly. Perform a superficial keratectomy to remove abnormal epithelium and fibrovascular pannus. Direct attention to donor eye and place a lid speculum in the donor eye. At the superior conjunctiva of the donor eye, measure and demarcate 6 mm at the limbus and extend 5–8 mm posterior from the limbus to create a trapezoid-shaped limbal graft. Inject 2 % lidocaine with epinephrine subconjunctivally in the superior conjunctiva to dissect away Tenon's capsule. Use Westcott scissors to transect the lateral and posterior margins of the graft and reflect the flap onto the cornea. Carefully dissect toward the cornea and extend through the palisades of Vogt to isolate the stem cells. Use Westcott scissors to transect the proximal margin and transfer graft to the donor eye. Maintain the correct epithelial and limbal orientation of the graft. Secure the graft with interrupted sutures using 10-0 nylon at the lateral margins and posterior margins. Do not place sutures through the limbal margin. Repeat the above steps to obtain the graft from the inferior limbus and the conjunctiva (Holland et al. 2011).

- Limbal stem cell transplantation via

> **Tip**
>
> Do not place sutures through the limbal margin.

living-related conjunctival limbal allograft (lr-CLAL)

Steps: lr-CLAL is a 2-operation surgical intervention. The first operation involves harvesting the allograft from the donor eye. The second operation involves transplanting the allograft onto the recipient eye. Anesthetize the donor eye with topical proparacaine eyedrops. Prep and drape the eye and place a lid speculum in the eye. At the superior conjunctiva of the donor eye, measure and demarcate 6 mm at the limbus and extend 5–8 mm posterior from the limbus to create a trapezoid-shaped limbal graft. Use gentian violet marker to make the marking asymmetric to help with reestablishing orientation during the transplantation surgery. Inject 2 % lidocaine with epinephrine subconjunctivally in the superior conjunctiva to dissect away Tenon's capsule. Use Westcott scissors to transect the lateral and posterior margins of the graft and reflect the flap onto the cornea. Carefully dissect toward the cornea and extend through the palisades of Vogt to isolate the stem cells. Use Westcott scissors to transect the proximal margin. Place the tissue on globe paper and immerse in colloidal storage solution for transfer to the recipient.

Anesthetize the recipient eye with topical proparacaine eyedrops. Prep and drape the eye and place a lid speculum in the eye. Inject 2 % lidocaine with epinephrine in the subconjunctival region. Perform a conjunctival peritomy of the recipient eye. Undermine the conjunctiva so it can recess posteriorly. Perform a superficial keratectomy to remove abnormal epithelium and fibrovascular pannus. Maintain the correct epithelial and limbal orientation of the graft. Secure the graft with interrupted sutures using 10-0 nylon at the lateral margins and posterior margins. Do not place sutures through the limbal margin. The allograft recipient will need to be on lifelong systemic immunosuppression, in addition to topical medications, for maintenance of graft survival (Holland et al. 2011).

- Limbal stem cell transplantation via keratolimbal allograft (KLAL)

Steps: Anesthetize the recipient eye with topical proparacaine eyedrops. Prep and drape the eye. Place a lid speculum in the recipient eye. If exposure is difficult because of superior and/or inferior symblepharon, a lateral canthotomy can be performed. Inject 2 % lidocaine with epinephrine in the subconjunctival region if possible. Severe scarring may limit this step. Perform a conjunctival 360° peritomy. If significant bleeding occurs, one quadrant can be resected at a time. Wetfield cautery, thrombin, and topical epinephrine (1:10,000 dilution) can be used to maintain hemostasis. Undermine the conjunctiva so it can recess posteriorly. Resect the conjunctiva 4–5 mm from the limbus to expose an area of sclera bed for the KLAL tissue. Avoid excising the symblepharon in the fornices, as this may result in a large epithelial defect on the palpebral conjunctiva side and exacerbate symblepharon formation postoperatively. Perform a superficial keratectomy to remove abnormal epithelium and fibrovascular pannus.

Attention is directed toward the cadaveric donor tissue. Use a 7.5-mm trephine to obtain the corneoscleral rim by excising the central cornea of the donor tissue in a similar manner as trephination performed for cutting a corneal button in routine keratoplasty. Section the corneoscleral rim into equal halves. Use Westcott scissors to trim off the excess peripheral scleral tissue, leaving 1mm of sclera peripheral to the limbus. Use a crescent blade to perform lamellar dissection to the posterior 1/2–2/3 of each hemisection to remove the posterior sclera and posterior stroma, including Descemet's membrane and endothelial stroma.

Repeat the above steps for the second half of the corneoscleral tissue and for the second donor tissue. A total of four halves of corneoscleral rims (two from each donor tissue) are needed for each recipient eye in order to have no gaps in the recipient limbus. Place the four corneoscleral crescent halves epithelial side up in storage medium while awaiting transplantation onto the recipient eye. Place two of the corneoscleral crescent halves on the recipient's eye in the correct orientation, with the cornea edges just overlying the recipient limbus.

Secure the anterior corners of each crescent half at the limbus with interrupted 10-0 nylon sutures, with the corneal edge of the KLAL laying flush to the recipient cornea. Additional sutures can be placed along the posterior edge for additional security. Additional crescents are added and placed flush with the previously placed crescents, as well as with the recipient cornea, until the entire limbus is covered circumferentially. The additional crescents may need to be trimmed in length to provide adequate apposition. The free edges of the previously recessed recipient conjunctiva are then sutured to the posterior edges of the crescents. Place an eye patch and an eye shield over the eye until postoperative appointment. The allograft recipient will need to be on lifelong systemic immunosuppression, in addition to topical medications, for maintenance of graft survival (Holland et al. 2011).

- Limbal stem cell transplantation via combined conjunctival limbal and keratolimbal allograft (C-KLAL)

Steps: Anesthetize the donor eye with topical proparacaine eyedrops. Prep and drape the eye and place a lid speculum in the eye. At the superior conjunctiva of the donor eye, measure and demarcate 6 mm at the limbus and extend 5–8 mm posterior from the limbus to create a trapezoid-shaped limbal graft. Use gentian violet marker to make the marking asymmetric to help with reestablishing orientation during the transplantation surgery. Inject 2 % lidocaine with epinephrine subconjunctivally in the superior conjunctiva to dissect away Tenon's capsule.

Use Westcott scissors to transect the lateral and posterior margins of the graft and reflect the flap onto the cornea. Carefully dissect toward the cornea and extend through the palisades of Vogt to isolate the stem cells. Use Westcott scissors to transect the proximal margin. Place the tissue on globe paper and immerse in colloidal storage solution for transfer to the recipient.

Attention is turned toward the cadaveric donor tissue. Use a 7.5-mm trephine to obtain the corneoscleral rim by excising the central cornea of the donor tissue in a similar manner as trephination performed for cutting a corneal button in routine keratoplasty. Section the corneoscleral rim into equal halves. Use Westcott scissors to trim off the excess peripheral scleral tissue, leaving 1 mm of sclera peripheral to the limbus. Use a crescent blade to perform lamellar dissection to the posterior 1/2–2/3 of each hemisection to remove the posterior sclera and posterior stroma, including Descemet's membrane and endothelial stroma. Place the two corneoscleral crescent halves epithelial side up in storage medium while awaiting transplantation onto the recipient eye.

Anesthetize the recipient eye with topical proparacaine eyedrops. Prep and drape the eye and place a lid speculum in the recipient eye. If exposure is difficult because of superior and/or inferior symblepharon, a lateral canthotomy can be performed. Inject 2 % lidocaine with epinephrine in the subconjunctival region if possible. Severe scarring may limit this step. If conjunctiva is present, perform a conjunctival 360° peritomy. Try to preserve as much conjunctiva as possible. Wetfield cautery, thrombin, and topical epinephrine (1:10,000 dilution) can be used to maintain hemostasis. Undermine the conjunctiva so it can recess posteriorly. Avoid excising the symblepharon in the fornices, as this may result in a large epithelial defect on the palpebral conjunctiva side and exacerbate symblepharon formation postoperatively.

Perform a superficial keratectomy to remove abnormal epithelium and fibrovascular pannus. Place the conjunctival limbal allografts superiorly and inferiorly (at the 12 o'clock and 6 o'clock positions) and secure with interrupted sutures using 10-0 nylon at the lateral and posterior aspects of the grafts. Place the cadaveric corneoscleral crescents at the temporal and nasal limbus and secure with interrupted sutures using 10-0 nylon at the anterior and posterior edges of the crescents. If needed, a symblepharon ring can be placed to maintain the fornices during the period of ocular surface re-epithelialization. The allograft recipient will need to be on lifelong systemic immunosuppression, in addition to topical medications, for maintenance of graft survival (Holland et al. 2011).

6.5 Summary

The surgical intervention for dry eyes should be guided and categorized by the primary etiology of the symptoms. These categories include **tear volume underproduction, tear film instability, mechanical disturbance, and ocular surface damage**. In tear volume underproduction, choose surgical approaches which extend the amount of time tears remain on the ocular surface by blocking or narrowing the tear drainage system. In tear film instability, plugged and dysfunctioning meibomian glands are usually the culprit, and interventions which restore functionality of these glands greatly enhance patients' dry eye symptoms. Mechanical disturbances can be secondary to conjunctivochalasis, lower eyelid malpositions, or eyelid dysfunctions. Surgically addressing the correct problem will resolve the dry eye symptoms. In ocular surface damage, oftentimes the damage is so severe that the cornea cannot repair itself due to destruction of the limbal cell population. Surgical approaches to this problem often involve allografts and lifelong systemic immunosuppression. Only when the correct category of a case of dry eyes is identified, can one choose the appropriate surgical technique to fix the problem and help the patient.

Compliance with Ethical Requirements Lingo Y. Lai, Clark L. Springs, and Richard A. Burgett declare they have no conflict of interest. No animal or human studies were carried out by the authors for this chapter.

References

Anderson RL, Gordy DD (1979) The tarsal strip procedure. Arch Ophthalmol 97(11):2192–2196

Chun YS, Park IK, Kim JC (2011) Technique for autologous nasal mucosa transplantation in severe ocular disease. Eur J Ophthalmol 21(5):545–551

Doss LR, Doss EL, Doss RP (2012) Paste-pinch-cut conjunctivoplasty: subconjunctival fibrin sealant injection in the repair of conjunctivochalasis. Cornea 31(8):959–962

Dresner SC, Karesh JW (1993) Transconjunctival entropion repair. Arch Ophthalmol 111:1144–1149

Georgiadis NS, Terzidou CD (2001) Epiphora caused by conjunctivochalasis. Cornea 20(6):619–621

Greiner JV (2012) A single Lipiflow thermal pulsation system treatment improves meibomian gland dysfunction and reduces dry eye symptoms for nine months. Curr Eye Res 37(4):272–278

Güerrissi JO, Belmonte J (2004) Surgical treatment of dry eye syndrome: conjunctival graft of the minor salivary gland. J Craniofac Surg 15(1):6–10

Hara S, Kojima T, Ishida R, Goto E, Matsumoto Y, Kaido M, Shimazaki J, Dogru M, Tsubota K (2011) Evaluation of tear stability after surgery for conjunctivochalasis. Optom Vis Sci 88(9):1112–1118

Holland EJ, Schwartz GS, Daya SM, Djalilian A (2011) Surgical techniques for ocular surface reconstruction. In: Krachmer JH, Mannis MJ, Holland EJ (eds) Cornea, vol 2, 3rd edn. Elsevier, St. Louis, pp 1727–1744

Holzchuh R, Villa Albers MB, Osaki TH, Igami TZ, Santo RM, Kara-Jose N, Holzchuh N, Hida RY (2011) Two-year outcome of partial lacrimal punctal occlusion in the management of dry eye related to Sjögren's syndrome. Curr Eye Res 36(6):507–512

Jacobsen H, Hakim SG, Trenkle T, Nitschke M, Steven P, Sieg P (2013) Allogeneic submandibular gland transplantation following hematopoietic stem cell transplantation. J Craniomaxillofac Surg 41(8):764–769

Kheirkhah A, Casas V, Blanco G, Li W, Hayashida Y, Chen Y, Tseng SCG (2007) Amniotic membrane transplantation with fibrin glue for conjunctivochalasis. Am J Ophthalmol 144:311–313

Kitchens J, Kinder J, Oetting T (2002) The drawstring temporary tarsorrhaphy technique. Arch Ophthalmol 120(2):187–190

Kronish JW (2001) Entropion. In: Chen WP (ed) Oculoplastic surgery. The Essentials Thieme, New York, pp 41–54

Lane SS, DuBiner HB, Epstein RJ, Ernest PH, Greiner JV, Hardten DR, Holland EJ, Lemp MA, McDonald JE, Silbert DI, Blackie CA, Stevens CA, Bedi R (2012) A new system, the Lipiflow, for the treatment of meibomian gland dysfunction (MGD). Cornea 31(4): 396–404

Liu D, Sadhan Y (2002) Surgical punctal occlusion: a prospective study. Br J Ophthalmol 86:1031–1034

Maskin S (2010) Intraductal meibomian gland probing relieves symptoms of obstructive meibomian gland dysfunction. Cornea 29(10):1145–1152

Muqit MMK, Ellingham RB, Daniel C (2007) Technique of amniotic membrane transplant dressing in the management of acute Stevens-Johnson syndrome. Br J Ophthalmol 91:1536

Ohba E, Dogru M, Hosaka E, Yamazaki A, Asaga R, Tatematsu Y, Ogawa Y, Tsubota K, Goto E (2011) Surgical punctal occlusion with a high heat-energy releasing cautery device for severe dry eye with recurrent punctal plug extrusion. Am J Ophthalmol 151(3):483–487

Otaka I, Kyu N (2000) A new surgical technique for management of conjunctivochalasis. Am J Ophthalmol 129:385–387

Sotozono C, Inatomi T, Nakamura T, Koizumi N, Yokoi N, Ueta M, Matsuyama K, Miyakoda K, Kaneda H, Fukushima M, Kinoshita S (2013) Visual improvement after cultivated oral mucosal epithelial transplantation. Ophthalmology 120:193–200

Tse DT, Negg AG (2001) Ectropion. In: Chen WP (ed) Oculoplastic surgery. The Essentials Thieme, New York, pp 55–66

Vieira AC, Mannis MJ (2011) Conjunctival flaps. In: Krachmer JH, Mannis MJ, Holland EJ (eds) Cornea, vol 2, 3rd edn. Elsevier, St. Louis, pp 1639–1645

Wang S, Ke M, Cai X, Chen X, Yu A, Dai H, Wen X (2012) An improved surgical method to correct conjunctivochalasis: conjunctival semiperitomy based on corneal limbus with subconjunctival cauterization. Can J Ophthalmol 47:418–422

Wladis EJ (2012) Intraductal meibomian gland probing in the management of ocular rosacea. Ophthal Plast Reconstr Surg 28(6):416–418

Dry Eye: Future Directions and Research

7

Minako Kaido and Kazuo Tsubota

7.1 Dry Eye Disease Demonstrates an Upward Trend

> **Causes for Dry Eye Occurrence**
> - Dryness: global warming, VDT work, and contact lens wear
> - Deterioration of the environment: smoking and infestation of chemicals and free radicals
> - Stressful society
> - Aging

Dry eye disease is prevalent. The upward trend of dry eye disease may be induced by recent environmental and lifestyle changes.

As its name suggests, dry eye is induced by dryness. Warming of the Earth's temperature accompanied by increasing desiccation, increasing *video display terminal* (*VDT*) *work* in a computer-controlled society, and contact lens wearing are risk factors for dry eye. Deterioration of the environment, such as *smoking* and infestation of *chemicals* and *free radicals*, is one of the risk factors for oxidative stress, which induces keratoconjunctival inflammation causing dry eye (Horwath-Winter et al. 2005; Augustin et al. 1995; Debbasch et al. 2000; Versura et al. 1999; Horwath and Schmut 2000). The involvement of the autonomic nerve system may be also an important factor in the mechanism for the occurrence of dry eye. Stressful society acts counter the parasympathetic nerve system, by which tear secretion is regulated.

Aging is also a risk factor for inducing dry eye. Dry eye disease may be regarded as an age-related disease, common in the elderly population (Schein et al. 1997; Moss et al. 2000; Schaumberg et al. 2003, 2009; Chia et al. 2003; Lin et al. 2003; Uchino et al. 2006; Viso et al. 2009). The aging of society has accelerated in recent decades. The elderly population in the United States aged 65 years or older has more than tripled in the past century (Haegerstrom-Portnoy et al. 1999). Lie et al. show a prevalence rate of 35 % of dry eye disease in Taiwan (Lin et al. 2003). A recent population-based data on dry eye disease in Japan, using self-diagnostic questionnaires and objective examinations in Japanese elderly subjects, revealed that, according to Japanese dry eye diagnostic criteria, 73.5 % of the eyes among elderly pensioners over 60 years had definite dry eyes (Uchino et al. 2006).

M. Kaido, MD, PhD (✉) • K. Tsubota, MD
Department of Ophthalmology, Keio University School of Medicine, 35 Shinanomachi, Shinjuku-ku, Tokyo 160-8582, Japan
e-mail: fwiw1193@mb.infoweb.ne.jp; tsubota@z3.keio.jp

C. Chan (ed.), *Dry Eye: A Practical Approach*, Essentials in Ophthalmology, DOI 10.1007/978-3-662-44106-0_7, © Springer-Verlag Berlin Heidelberg 2015

7.1.1 Focus on Aging

Aging is a risk factor for the dysfunction of organs in the body. Two main categories, programmed and error theories, have been proposed to explain the process of aging, but neither of them appears to be fully satisfactory (Zimniak 2008; Kunlin 2010). Recent newer concepts are *oxidative stress* and *metabolic syndrome*, which play a major role in the aging process (Fig. 7.1) (Harman 1956; Frisard and Ravussin 2006; Matsuzawa 2006).

The free radical theory: Generation of reactive oxygen species (ROS) eventually overwhelms the counteracting antioxidant defenses leading to cellular damage and aging.

The metabolic theory: Overeating creates *metabolic stress* on the body, which can lead to a shorter life span and serious age-related diseases.

7.1.2 Lacrimal Gland Change with Age

Aging is an important risk factor of dry eye. Age-related changes in the lacrimal gland are associated with alterations in the structural organization and functional response in the lacrimal gland (Damato et al. 1984; Sullivan et al. 1990; Obata et al. 1995). These changes include increased acinar atrophy, periductal

fibrosis and accumulation of lipofuscin-like inclusions, and an increase in inflammatory infiltrates, which contain mast cells and lymphocytes (Damato et al. 1984; Obata et al. 1995; Williams et al. 1994; Draper et al. 1998; Ríos et al. 2005):

- Histopathological change
  Acinar cell atrophy
  Fibrosis
  Ductal dilation
  Infiltration
  Accumulation of lipofuscin
- Lacrimal gland hypofunction
  Expanded acinar cells
  Accumulated enlarged secretory vesicle in the cytoplasm
  Decreased endoplasmic reticulum
  Increase in the nuclei with dark nucleoplasm

7.2 New Perspective on Dry Eye Diagnosis

The two major etiological causes of dry eye are aqueous tear-deficient dry eye and evaporative dry eye:

- Aqueous tear-deficient dry eye
- Evaporative dry eye (short BUT dry eye)

7.2.1 Aqueous Tear-Deficient Dry Eye

Aqueous-deficient dry eye is mainly caused by disorders of the lacrimal gland and occurs in Sjögren's syndrome–type and non-Sjögren's syndrome–type dry eye. Aqueous-deficient dry eye has two major groupings, Sjögren's syndrome dry eye and non-Sjögren's syndrome dry eye. Sjögren's syndrome–type dry eye results from

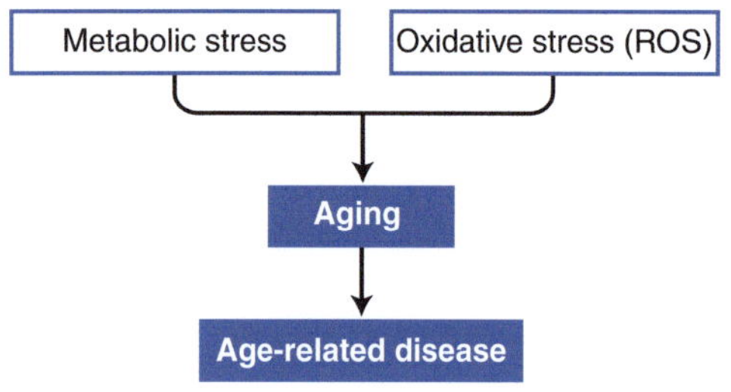

Fig. 7.1 Concept of aging

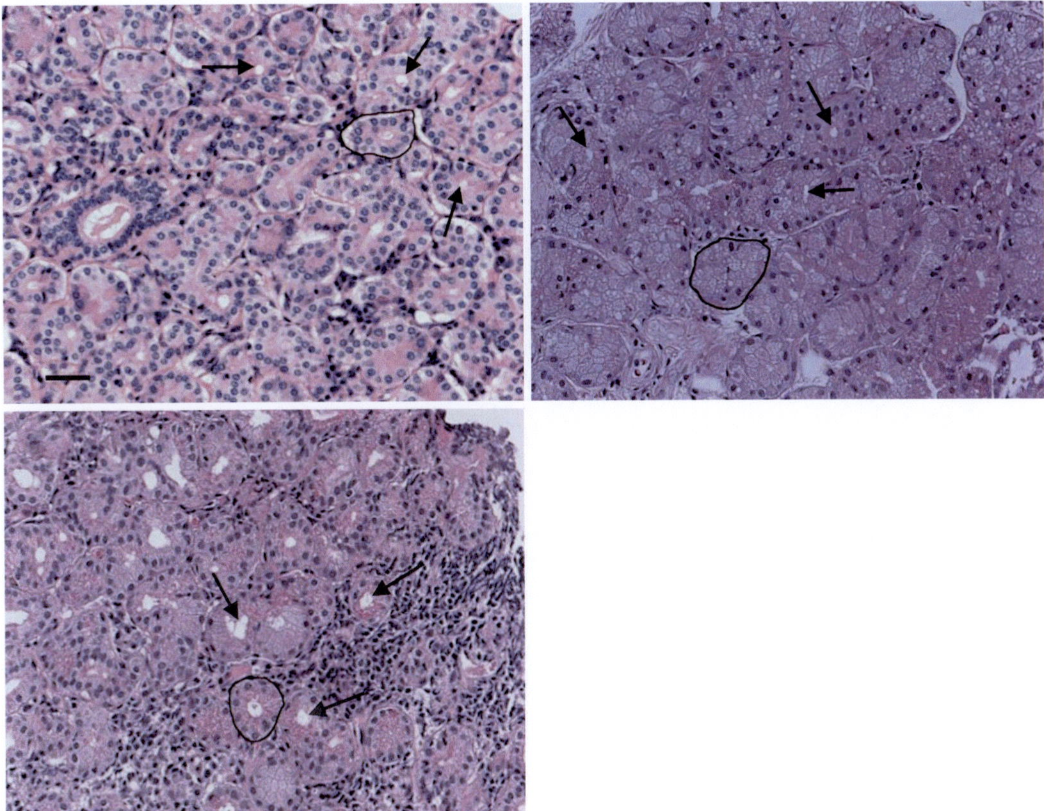

Fig. 7.2 An excessive secretory vesicle accumulation. H&E staining of lacrimal gland. (**a**) Normal control. The lacrimal gland structure consists of normal acinar cells, ductal cells, capillaries, and connective tissue. (**b**) Dry eye patient with VDT work. The lacrimal gland acini are larger than those in normal controls and show ductal obstruction. (**c**) Dry eye patient with Sjögren's syndrome. The destruction of acini with lymphocytic infiltration and ductal dilation are shown. *Arrows*: ductal lumens. *Circle*: one acinus. Scale bars = 50 mm (Reprinted with permission from Kamoi et al. (2012))

destruction of the lacrimal gland by lymphocytic infiltration and often induces severe epithelial damage.

One increasingly recognized version of non-Sjögren's syndrome dry eye may be caused by work involving the use of VDTs (visual display terminals/computer screens). VDT has been increasing with the development of information technology in the office environment and daily life. Many computer users suffer from dry eye related to VDT work. One of the causes for VDT-related dry eye is a decreased blinking frequency inducing the excessive evaporation of tear fluid (Tsubota and Nakamori 1993, 1995; Acosta et al. 1999; Kojima et al. 2011; Tsubota et al. 1996). Another cause may be lacrimal gland *hypofunction* (Nakamura et al. 2010; Kamoi et al. 2012). The mechanism of VDT-related dry eye was recently revealed showing that *excessive secretory vesicle accumulation* in the acinar epithelia resulting from the decreased blink frequency in VDT users may induce a failure of tear secretion (Figs. 7.2 and 7.3). There is a negative relationship between VDT use duration and tear secretion. Characteristically, working long hours using a VDT for many years may be a risk factor for inducing non-SS dry eye among VDT users. A new type of dry eye, lacrimal gland hypofunction, is advocated as a dry eye mechanism.

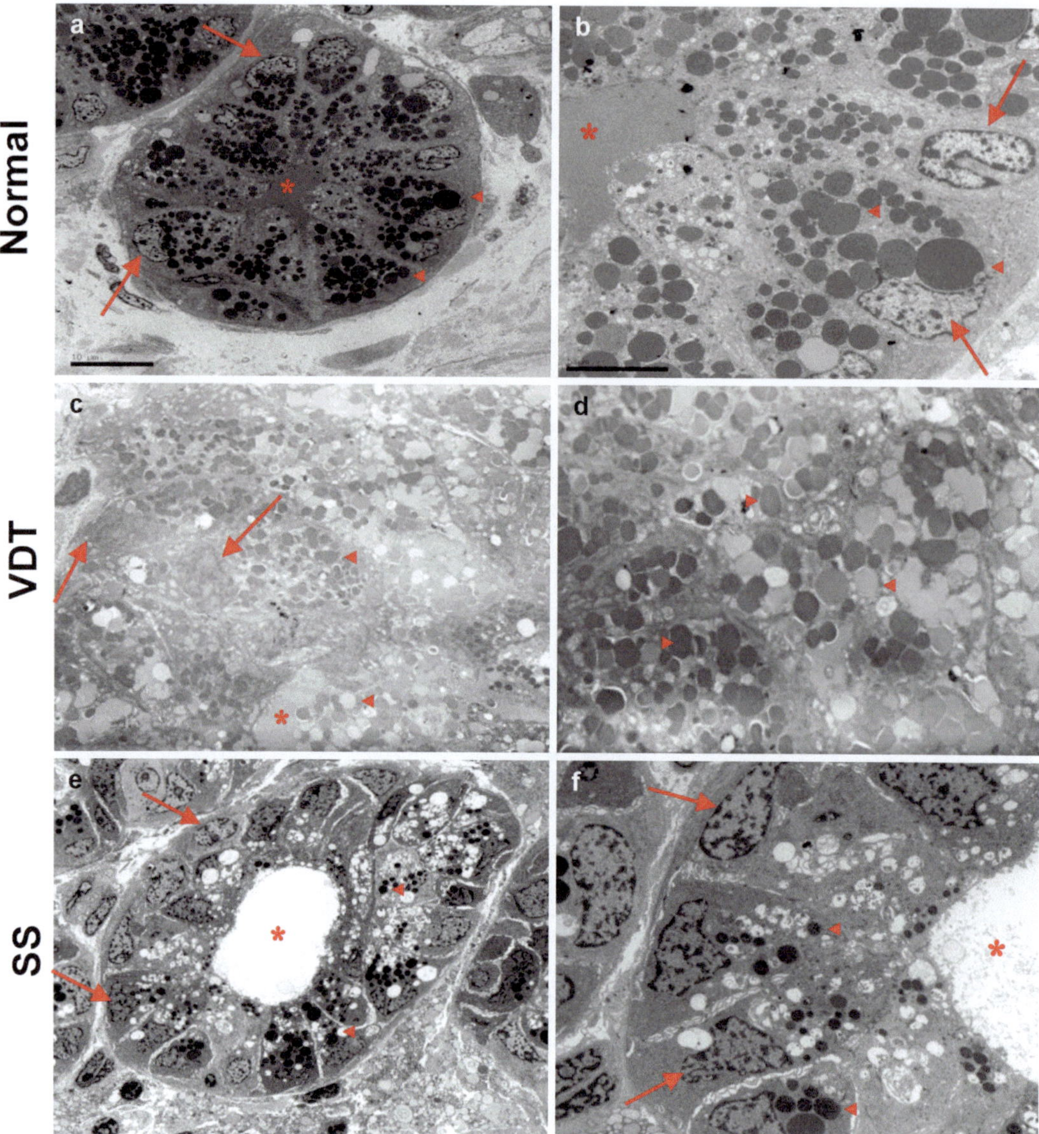

Fig. 7.3 Electron microscopic findings of the lacrimal gland. (**a**) Secretory vesicle (SV) accumulation in the normal. Scale bars = 10 mm. (**b**) Homogeneous SVs in normal controls. Scale bars = 5 mm (**a, b**) Show that SVs accumulated homogeneously toward the apical region of the lacrimal gland epithelial cells. (**c**) Excessive accumulation of SVs in the VDT group. (**d**) High-magnification view of SVs in the VDT group. (**c, d**) Show excessive accumulation of SVs and the nuclei displaced toward the cell periphery by the SVs, which filled the cytoplasm, in the VDT group. SVs of both high and low electron density are observed. (**e**) Only a few SVs in the SS group. (**f**) High-magnification view of SVs in the SS group. Figures (**e, f**) show only a few SVs and dilation of the duct. The SVs are also smaller than those in the normal and VDT groups. The TEM findings indicate that the VDT group has an unusually large number of SVs in the cytoplasm of the lacrimal gland epithelial cells compared with the other two groups. Original magnification: 62,000 (**a, c, e**), 65,000 (**b, d, f**). *Asterisk*, ductal lumen; *Arrows*, nuclei; triangle, SV (Reprinted with permission from Kamoi et al. (2012))

VDT/computer may be caused by lacrimal gland hypofunction due to reduced blink frequency.

7.2.2 Evaporative Dry Eye

Evaporative dry eye, which is the so-called short breakup time (BUT) dry eye, is characterized by excessive evaporation of the tear film layer from the ocular surface, while tear secretion is normal. Two major BUT patterns have been observed: one is a dry round spot pattern, and the other is a longitudinal tear break pattern (Fig. 7.4). It is sometimes misunderstood that short BUT dry eye represents an early milder form of dry eye, since it is associated with little or no corneal epithelial damage (Sullivan et al. 2010, 2012; Lemp et al. 2011). However, short BUT dry eye is strongly symptomatic. Dry eye symptoms may present as eye fatigue, discomfort, or heaviness but also as visual blur or discomfort during daily activities due to the impaired stability and regularity of tear film, despite a normal tear volume and the absence of corneal staining (Toda et al. 1993; Montes-Mico et al. 2004; Ridder et al. 2005, 2011; Goto et al. 2006; Tong et al. 2010; Walker et al. 2010; Koh et al. 2008; Kaido et al. 2012a).

It seems that short BUT dry eye patients have increased recently in office workers who perform *VDT work* and wear *contact lenses*. The etiology has been classified as intrinsic causes (*meibomian gland dysfunction (MGD)*, disorders of lid aperture, low blink rate) or extrinsic causes (vitamin A deficiency; topical drug preservatives, such as benzalkonium chloride (BAC); contact lens wear; and ocular surface disease, e.g., allergy) (Smith et al. 2007). One of the etiological explanations for the short BUT may be decreased goblet cell density (Toda et al. 1993, 1995; Watanabe 2002).

Short tear breakup time dry eye/evaporative tear loss is a major cause of dry eye in office workers. Loss of goblet cells may be an important factor.

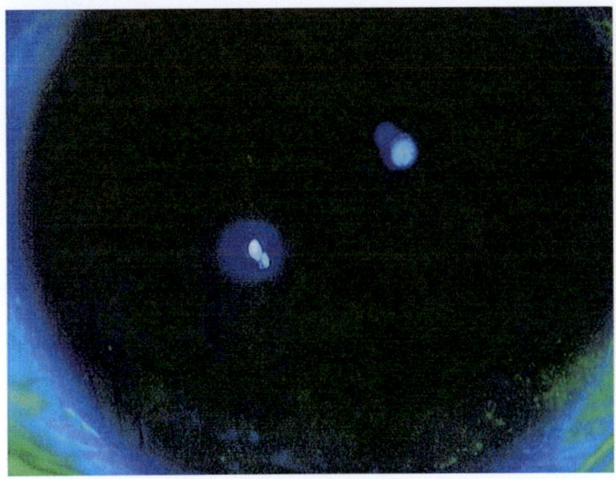

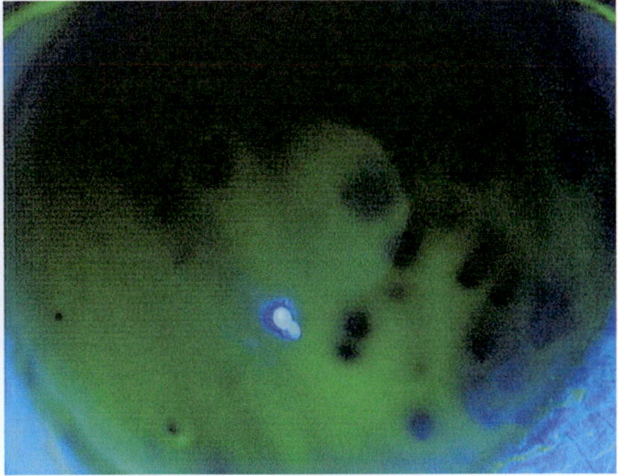

Fig. 7.4 Tear film breakup patterns. *Left*: Longitudinal tear break pattern is typically observed in elder females. *Right*: Round spot tear break pattern, which is observed equally in young males and females, may be related to allergic conjunctivitis and VDT work

7.3 New Examinations for the Tear Function Assessment

- Strip meniscometry
- TearLab Osmolarity
- Oily layer assessment: DR-1
- Functional visual acuity measurement system

7.3.1 Strip Meniscometry

Several methods are used for the assessment of dry eye diseases, including the Schirmer test, invasive and noninvasive tear film breakup time assessment, vital stainings, and tear meniscus evaluation. The Schirmer test is an indispensable tool for tear volume assessment; however, there is wide intrasubject and time-wise variability, as well as problems of irritation and induction of reflex tearing.

Strip meniscometry (SM) is a novel, simple, noninvasive method for measuring the tear meniscus volume (Dogru et al. 2006; Ibrahim et al. 2011). It is designed to avoid induction of reflex tearing and is promoted to be mechanically produced with high quality. The strip is applied to the lateral lower lid tear meniscus without touching the ocular surface for 5 s. The length of the stained tear column in the central membrane ditch is regarded as the SM value (Fig. 7.5).

The strip is composed of polyethylene terephthalate, on which is pasted a urethane-based material of the same size containing a central ditch of 0.40 mm in depth. A nitrocellulose membrane filter paper strip with a pore size of 8 μm impregnated in natural blue dye is then placed into the central ditch.

The SM has a strong correlation with the Schirmer test, BUT, ocular surface vital staining scores, and tear film lipid layer interferometry grades. It is noted that sensitivity and specificity for dry eye diagnosis are high, such as 80.5 and 67.2 % using a single SM, and elevated to 80.5

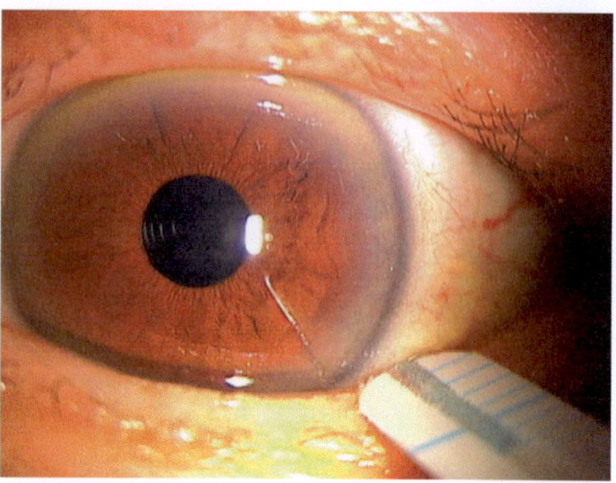

Fig. 7.5 Strip meniscometry. The strip is applied to the lateral lower lid tear meniscus without touching the ocular surface. Length of the stained tear column in the central membrane ditch is regarded as the strip meniscometry value

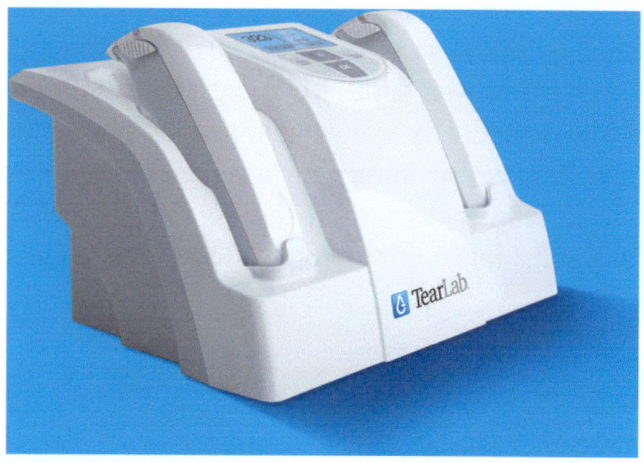

Fig. 7.6 TearLab Osmolarity (Courtesy of TearLab Corp., San Diego, CA)

and 99.3 % using SM and BUT values (Ibrahim et al. 2011).

7.3.2 TearLab Osmolarity

The *TearLab Osmolarity System* is the first objective and quantitative test for diagnosing and managing dry eye patients (Lemp and Foulks 2007; Nichols and Sinnott 2006; Lemp et al. 2013). The TearLab Osmolarity System is intended to measure the osmolarity of human tears to aid in the diagnosis of patients suspected of having dry eye disease, in conjunction with other methods of clinical evaluation

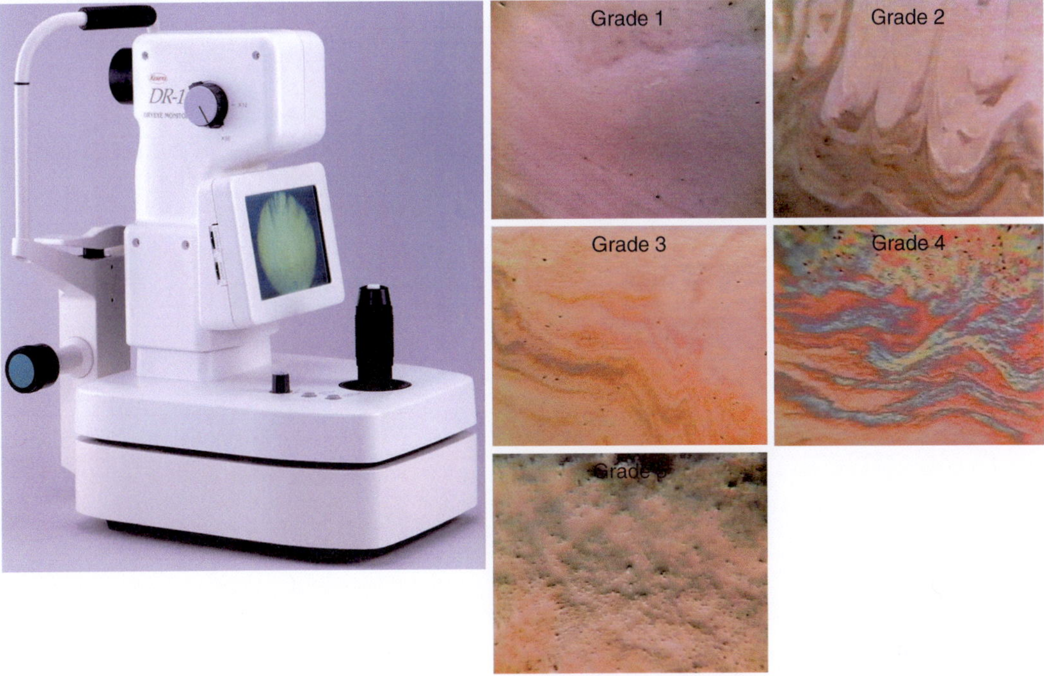

Fig. 7.7 The DR-1 images (Courtesy of Norihiko Yokoi, Kyoto Prefectural University of Medicine)

(Fig. 7.6). Hyperosmolarity has been described in the literature as a primary marker of tear film integrity. When the quantity or quality of secreted tears is compromised, increased rates of evaporation lead to a more concentrated tear film (increased osmolarity) that places stress on the corneal epithelium and conjunctiva. The system has been shown to correctly identify 88 % of normal tear subjects, 75 % of mild-to-moderate dry eye disease subjects, and 95 % of severe dry eye disease subjects (Lemp and Foulks 2007).

7.3.3 DR-1

The DR-1 device (Kowa Co., Nagoya, Japan) is the specific interference camera to visualize the precorneal lipid layer spread (Goto et al. 2003). The interference color chart allows quantification of the interference images, which are graded corresponding to dry eye severity. The DR-1 images were classified from grades 1–5 as follows: grade 1, somewhat gray color and uniform distribution; grade 2, somewhat gray color and nonuniform distribution; grade 3, a few colors and nonuniform distribution; grade 4, many colors and nonuniform distribution; and grade 5, corneal surface partially exposed (Fig. 7.7). It is noted that the severity of dryness on the ocular surface and meibomian gland dysfunction is related to the grades of interference patterns.

DR-1 Grading Scores
Grade 1—somewhat gray color and uniform distribution
Grade 2—somewhat gray color and nonuniform distribution
Grade 3—a few colors and nonuniform distribution
Grade 4—many colors and nonuniform distribution
Grade 5—corneal surface partially exposed

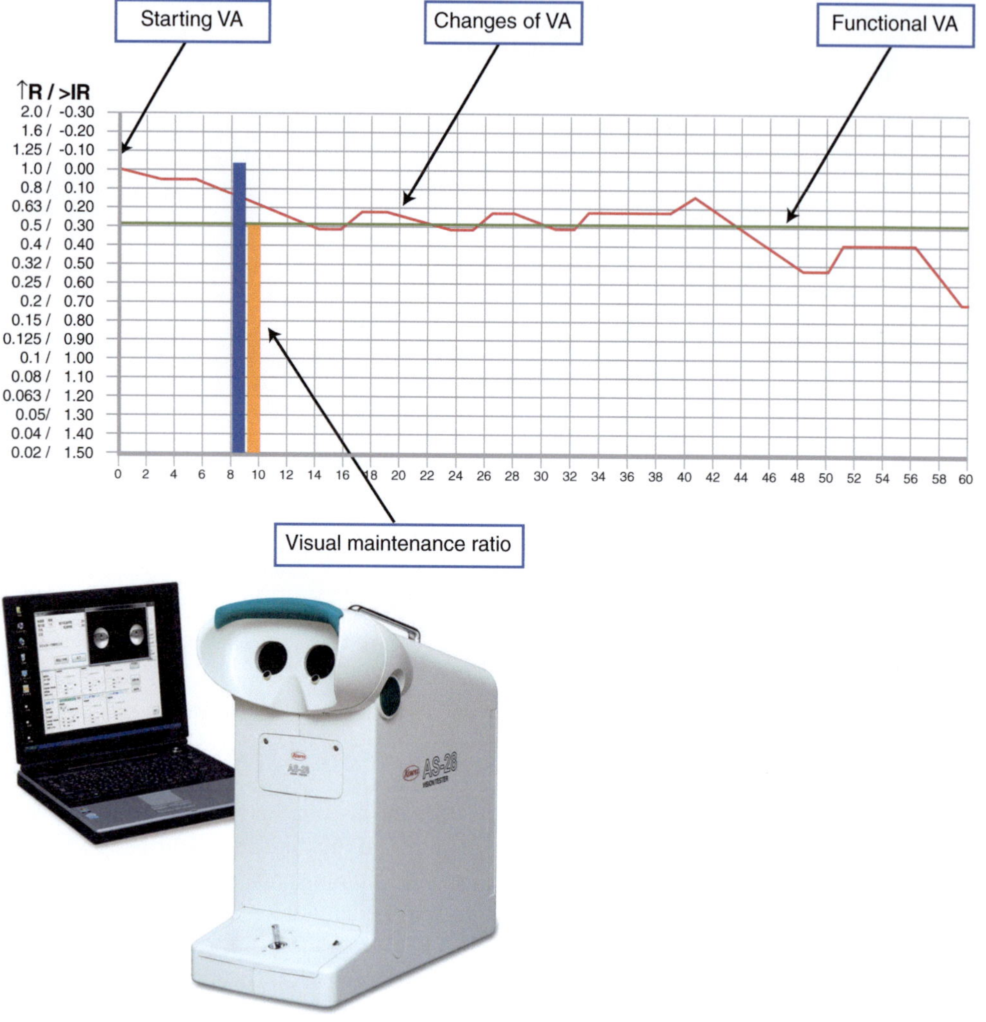

Fig. 7.8 Functional visual acuity measurement system. *Upper*: functional visual acuity measurement system (Kowa Co., Nagoya, Japan). *Lower*: the sequential changes in visual acuity over time

7.3.4 Functional Visual Acuity Measurement System

The 2007 International Dry Eye Workshop Epidemiology Subcommittee recommended inclusion of an item on visual function in the definition of dry eye——including fluctuation of vision or transient blurred vision——to capture the effect of ocular surface dryness on visual function and assist in defining a clinically meaningful situation (Smith et al. 2007). Standard visual acuity testing measures instantaneous visual acuity and has been traditionally accepted for assessing the visual function; however, standard testing may have limitations to assess the quality of vision. Several methods, such as contrast sensitivity, corneal topography, glare test, wavefront sensor, and functional visual acuity measurement system, have been developed to assess the quality of an individual's visual acuity.

Functional visual acuity measurement system (Kowa Co., Nagoya, Japan) is a device that examines the change in visual acuity over time (Fig. 7.8). Functional VA is an index of mean VA value over time. A stable tear film over the corneal surface is essential for clear visual imaging, and an irregular corneal surface resulting from dry eyes is associated with poor quality of vision. Functional visual acuity is effective in evaluating dynamic visual function changes relating with tear film (Ishida et al. 2005; Kaido et al. 2011, 2012a, b).

> **Index of Functional Visual Acuity Measurement**
> 1. *Starting visual acuity*: baseline visual acuity starting with best corrected visual acuity
> 2. *Functional visual acuity*: the mean VA score of only the correct responses during the measurement period
> 3. *Visual maintenance ratio*: the ratio of functional VA divided by the value of baseline VA
> 4. *Maximal visual acuity*: the highest visual acuity during the measurement period
> 5. *Minimal visual acuity*: the lowest VA score during the measurement period
> 6. *Response reaction time*
> 7. *Blink frequency*

7.4 Dry Eye Treatments

7.4.1 New Equipment for Dry Eye Treatments

JINS Moisture glasses are designed for the protection of the eyes from dryness. These have a small container filled with water on the side (Fig. 7.9). The moisture glasses are suitable for anyone who suffers from severe eye pain due to dryness but also experiences the irritation that comes with sitting in front of a computer screen for a few hours.

7.4.2 Dry Eye Treatments on Tear Film–Oriented Therapy

Tear film–oriented therapy (TFOT) is a new strategic direction for treating dry eye. Tear film stability and regularity are based on the

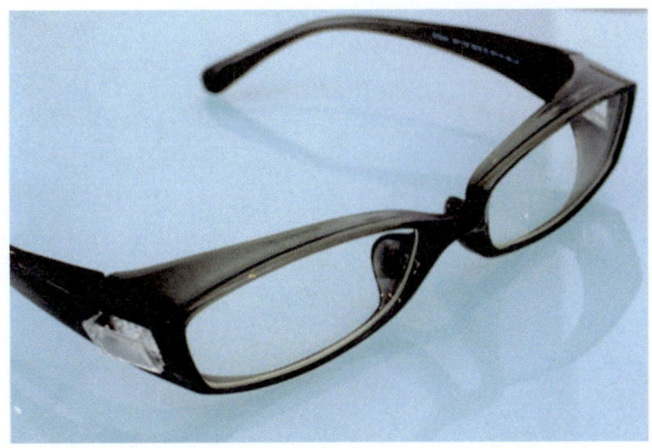

Fig. 7.9 JINS Moisture glasses

balance of the trilaminar tear film—consisting of lipid, aqueous, and mucin layers—on the ocular surface. Lipid meibom reduces aqueous evaporation. The lacrimal glands produce the tears that make up the aqueous layer, and mucins provide wettability and an intimate layer of protection at the corneal and conjunctival surface. The TFOT is the treatment targeting the specific tear layers on the ocular surface (Fig. 7.10).

> **New Eye Drops for Tear Film–Orientated Therapy (TFOT)**
> - Diquafosol tetrasodium ophthalmic solution
> - Rebamipide ophthalmic solution

7.4.3 Diquafosol Tetrasodium Ophthalmic Solution

Diquafosol tetrasodium, a P_2Y_2 receptor agonist, is a new preparation of eye drops that stimulates *tear and mucin secretion* which improves tear film stability (Fujihara et al. 2001, 2002; Takaoka-Shichijo and Nakamura 2011). The induction of mucin production from the ocular surface may increase the stability of the tear film. It is noted that the administration of diquafosol tetrasodium ophthalmic solution has beneficial effects on tear film stability and/or optical quality and on visual performance in short BUT dry eye (Kaido et al. 2013).

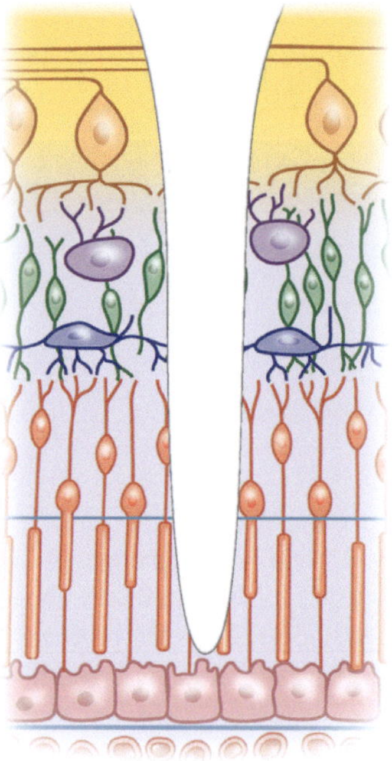

Target for therapy		Target eye therapy
	Lipid layer	Warm compress and lid hygiene Low-dose ophthalmic ointment Certain types of OTC *Diquafosol sodium
Aqueous /Mucous	Aqueous component	Artificial tears Sodium hyaluronate Diquafosol sodium Punctal plug
	Secretory mucin	Diquafosol sodium Rebamipide
Epithelium	Membrane associated mucins	Diquafosol sodium Rebamipide
	Epithelial cells (Goblet cell)	Autologous serum EGF (Rebamipide)
Ocular surface inflammation		Cyclosporin Steroids **Rebamipide

*Diquafosol sodium may increase the function of the tear film lipid layer by promoting speading of the lipid layer through lipid and tear fluid secretion.

**Rebarnipide may suppress the inflammation of the ocular surface in dry eye by its anti-inflammatory action.

Fig. 7.10 Tear film-oriented therapy (TFOT) (Courtesy of the Japanese Dry Eye Society)

7.4.4 Rebamipide Ophthalmic Suspension

Rebamipide, an amino acid derivative of 2(1H)-quinolinone, is originally a gastroprotective drug, which has been used for *mucosal protection, healing of gastroduodenal ulcers*, and *treatment of gastritis* (Uchida et al. 1985). Rebamipide suspension was then developed more recently for use in the ophthalmic field. The therapeutic effects of rebamipide demonstrate an increase in corneal and conjunctival mucin-like substances and improve corneal and conjunctival injury in vivo (Urashima et al. 2004). It is noted that rebamipide increased the mucin production in cultured conjunctival goblet cells and in corneal epithelial cells (Rios et al. 2006, 2008).

7.5 New Dry Eye Approach with Oral Supplements

New Approach on Oral Supplement
- Lactoferrin
- Omega-3 fatty acids

Tear lactoferrin level, which is *an indicator of lacrimal secretory function*, is decreased in dry eye (Danjo et al. 1994). Lacrimal gland secretory function is correlated with age-induced dry eye disease in rats, which may stem from oxidative stress; lactoferrin concentration in tears decreases with age (Jensen et al. 1986; McGill et al. 1984).

Lactoferrin has an *antioxidant* effect in that it binds free iron, thus preventing the production of hydroxyl radicals. Lactoferrin is also known to have an *anti-inflammatory* effect. The increased occurrence of eye surface infections and the uncontrolled development of inflammation typical of dry eye have been reported to be a result of the reduced amount of lactoferrin in the tear film (Baveye et al. 1999; Kanyshkova et al. 2001; Legrand et al. 2005).

It has been shown that *oral lactoferrin administration* preserves lacrimal gland function in aged mice by attenuating oxidative damage and suppressing subsequent gland inflammation (Kawashima et al. 2012). One report showed the improvement of tear stability and ocular surface damage in patients with Sjögren's syndrome by the oral lactoferrin supplementation (Dogru et al. 2007). Lactoferrin supplementation is expected to be a safe and effective therapy for age-related decline of lacrimal gland dysfunction by attenuating oxidative damage and suppressing subsequent gland inflammation.

Lactoferrin

- An iron-binding glycoprotein present in serum and exocrine secretions
- Anti-inflammatory effects
- The promotion of cell growth and DNA synthesis
- Exhibition of anti-angiogenic and anti-tumorigenic properties
- Antioxidative and carcinogenic bioactivities

7.5.1 Omega-3 Fatty Acids

Omega-3 fatty acids, including docosahexaenoic acid (DHA), eicosapentaenoic acid (EPA), and alpha-linolenic acid (ALA), cannot be synthesized by the human body but are vital for normal metabolism. DHA, the major polyunsaturated fatty acid found in retinal rod outer segments, is noted to play a role in the prevention of age-related macular degeneration and dry eye syndrome (Miljanović et al. 2005). Omega-3 essential fatty acids have *anti-inflammatory* effects and inhibit multiple aspects of inflammatory response as demonstrated in the lacrimal gland where omega-3s prevent apoptosis of the secretory epithelial cells. Supplementation is expected to clear meibomitis, allowing a thinner, more elastic lipid layer to protect the tear film and cornea and treat dry eye disease.

7.6 Dry Eye Treatments by an Antiaging Approach

Because dry eye is exacerbated by aging, a useful approach for the prevention or treatment of dry eye may be to interfere with the aging process.

Prevention of cellular oxidation and calorie restriction may slow or prevent aging and therefore dry eye.

Antiaging medicine may expand the possibilities for the dry eye treatments. Age-related changes in tears and lacrimal gland secretary function lead to an increased prevalence of dry eye disease (Moss et al. 2000; Schaumberg et al. 2003, 2009; Chia et al. 2003; Lin et al. 2003; Uchino et al. 2006; Viso et al. 2009). The aging process may be managed by controlling reactive oxygen species or levels of calories as an antiaging strategy (Harman 1956; Frisard and Ravussin 2006; Matsuzawa 2006). The two important antiaging strategies, prevention of cellular oxidation and calorie restriction, are examined, and how to apply these theories for the prevention and treatment of dry eye is discussed below.

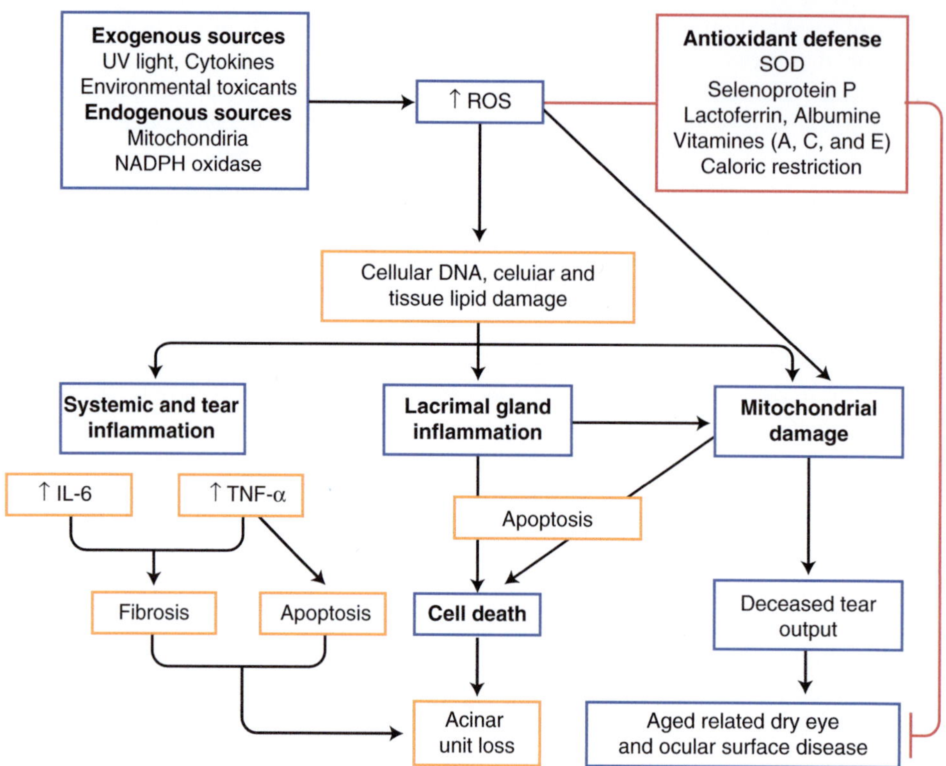

Fig. 7.11 Oxidative stress theory of dry eye

7.6.1 Prevention of Cellular Oxidation as an Antiaging Strategy

The *oxidative stress* theory has become increasingly accepted as part of the aging process. *Reactive oxygen species* (*ROS*), which primarily result from normal mitochondrial metabolism, cause progressive damage resulting in the functional decline that defines aging (Harman 1956). Oxidative stress is caused by an imbalance between the production of ROS and the ability of the biological systems' defense mechanism necessary to eliminate the stress. Oxidative stress is implicated in many acute and chronic diseases, even in several ocular diseases including age-related macular degeneration, cataract, uveitis, retinopathy of prematurity, corneal inflammation, and keratitis (Imamura et al. 2006; Spector 1995; Gritz et al. 1991; Niesman et al. 1997; Alio et al. 1995a, b).

An increased awareness of oxidative stress damage and its relation with ocular surface diseases has led to newly discovered mechanisms in the development of dry eye disease (Fig. 7.11). For example, superficial punctuate keratopathy (SPK) is accompanied by an increase of oxidative stress markers, the expression in antioxidant-related gene, and ROS production in corneal epithelia (Alio et al. 1995a). These findings suggest a strong relationship between the accumulation of oxidative stress and the etiology of corneal epithelial alterations in dry eye (Alio et al. 1995a; Nakamura et al. 2007). Both oxidative tissue damage and polymorphonuclear leukocytes indicating oxidative potential occur in the tear film of patients with dry eyes. These reactions lead to severe damage of the involved tissue. Free radicals and inflammation may be involved in the pathogenesis or in the self-propagation of the disease.

The toxic effect of these reactive oxygen species and free radicals can be eliminated by enzymes.

Some enzymes in the body prevent cellular oxidation, including *superoxide dismutase* (*SOD*) known for its powerful antioxidation reaction (Valentine et al. 2005). This finding raised the possibility that the supplements may prevent dry eye disease.

Selenoprotein P (SeP) is a carrier of selenium, which is an essential trace element for oxidative stress metabolism in the body, and is extremely expressed in lacrimal gland. Administration of SeP eye drops in a rat dry eye model, prepared by removing the lacrimal glands, induces the improvement in corneal dry eye index and the suppression of oxidative stress markers (Higuchi et al. 2010). Tear SeP is a key molecule to protect the ocular surface cells against environmental oxidative stress.

> Reducing oxidative stress by aiding the body's existing antioxidant mechanisms is a future direction for dry eye medications.

It is still unclear whether oxidative stress is the primary initiating event that is associated with some eye diseases. However, a growing body of evidence implicates it as being involved in at least the propagation of cellular injury that leads to eye pathology in these various conditions. It is biologically relevant in vivo and is intimately linked with an integrated series of cellular events. Interaction between these various components is not necessarily a cascade but might be a cycle of events, of which oxidative stress is a major component. Inhibition of oxidative stress therapeutically might act to "break the cycle" of cell death.

7.6.2 Calorie Restriction as an Antiaging Strategy

Caloric restriction (*CR*), which refers to curbing the dietary intake to 30–50 % less than the normal level calorie consumption, is the only scientifically proven strategy to prevent functional decline of various organs due to aging (Fig. 7.12) (Masoro 2000). CR profoundly affects the physiological and pathophysiological alterations associated with aging in several species, which delays the onset of numerous age-associated diseases including cancer, atherosclerosis, and diabetes (Spindler 2001; Blagosklonny 2007; Heilbronn et al. 2006). CR has been reported to decrease excessive ROS production in postmitotic tissues (Kawashima et al. 2010). Mitochondria are considered to be the most important cellular organelles as a source of ROS production (Paradies et al. 2010). Aging occurs, in part, as a result of the accumulation of oxidative stress status caused by ROS that are generated continuously during the course of metabolic processes. In the field of dry eye disease, CR could prevent age-related decline of lacrimal gland function and morphological changes by attenuating oxidative damage and inflammation in the lacrimal gland.

Sirtuins have been implicated in influencing aging and regulating transcription, apoptosis, and stress resistance (Guarente 2008; Longo and Kennedy 2006). CR induces the activation of sirtuin, resulting in various kinds of gene upregulation associated with longevity. CR affects gene expression patterns during aging and provides for a healthier life. Antiaging approach is applied to the prevention and treatment of age-related dry eye.

> Calorie restriction may cause upregulation of sirtuins, which may lengthen life span and reduce dry eye.

Resveratrol, a *polyphenol* found abundantly in red wines, grape skin, and peanut skin, among other food items, has the same effect as CR in lengthening life span, due to the activation of the sirtuin gene (Baur et al. 2006; Pearson et al. 2008). The strategy of using resveratrol for the treatment of dry eye is also appealing. It is expected that the resveratrol could increase the tear volume and also have an effect on suppression of inflammation of the lacrimal gland and the ocular surface in a dry eye. Because inflammation is considered a major contributing factor to the pathogenesis of dry eye, this may be a new

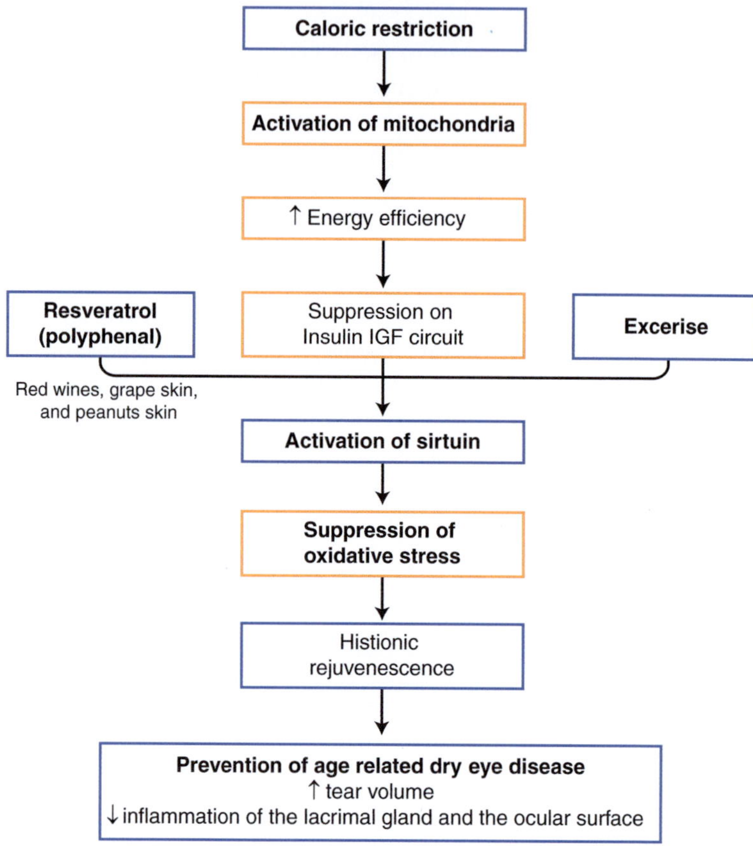

Fig. 7.12 Caloric restriction theory of dry eye

approach for the control of dry eye in addition to other treatments such as cyclosporine A or other anti-inflammatory agents.

In the clinical setting, there is no fundamental treatment available to increase tear secretion despite the robust increase in patients suffering from dry eye disease. Therefore, findings observed in the studies may have clinically significant implication in the field of ophthalmology. CR as a treatment modality may shed new light on the mechanism of age-related dry eye disease and provide a novel therapeutic strategy for treating patients with dry eyes.

7.7 Summary

Action against dysfunction, health impairment, and diseases induced by aging faces an urgent attention in aging societies. One of the age-related diseases, dry eye, tends to demonstrate an upward trend. Present trends raise the possibility of antiaging medicine accomplishing not only treatment of diseases but a healthier and longer life. Thus, intervention of the aging process may be a useful treatment of the age-related diseases. Further investigation is expected on the key regulators, such as gene expression analysis on understanding of the IGF/insulin signal pathway, mTOR pathway, sirtuins, and secretion-related molecules; tear composition on metabolome analysis; and proteome analysis. Dry eye can now be targeted by this approach, and elucidating the mechanism is currently underway. This approach opens up new therapeutic options for dry eye, and the future is promising.

Compliance with Ethical Requirements

Conflict of Interest Kazuo Tsubota is a consultant for Santen Pharmaceutical Co., Ltd.

Kazuo Tsubota has received research grants from Santen Pharmaceutical Co., Ltd.; Kowa Co., Ltd.; Otsuka Pharmaceutical Co., Ltd; and JIN Co., Ltd.

Kazuo Tsubota and Minako Kaido hold patent rights for the method and the apparatus used for the measurement of functional visual acuity (US patent no: 7470026).

Informed Consent All procedures followed were in accordance with the ethical standards of the responsible committee on human experimentation (institutional and national) and with the Helsinki Declaration of 1975, as revised in 2000 (5). Informed consent was obtained from all patients for being included in the study.

References

Acosta MC, Gallar J, Belmonte C (1999) The influence on eye solutions of blinking and ocular comfort at rest and during work at video display terminals. Exp Eye Res 68:663–669

Alio JL, Artola A, Serra A, Ayala MJ, Mulet ME (1995a) Effect of topical antioxidant therapy on experimental infectious keratitis. Cornea 14:175–179

Alio JL, Ayala MJ, Mulet ME, Artola A, Ruiz JM, Bellot J (1995b) Antioxidant therapy in the treatment of experimental acute corneal inflammation. Ophthalmic Res 27:136–143

Augustin AJ, Spitznas M, Kaviani N, Meller D, Koch FH, Grus F, Göbbels MJ (1995) Oxidative reactions in the tear fluid of patients suffering from dry eyes. Graefes Arch Clin Exp Ophthalmol 233:694–698

Baur JA, Pearson KJ, Price NL et al (2006) Resveratrol improves health and survival of mice on a high-calorie diet. Nature 444:337–342

Baveye S, Elass E, Mazurier J, Spik G, Legrand D (1999) Lactoferrin: a multifunctional glycoprotein involved in the modulation of the inflammatory process. Clin Chem Lab Med 37:281–286

Blagosklonny MV (2007) An anti-aging drug today: from senescence-promoting genes to anti-aging pill. Drug Discov Today 12:218–224

Chia EM, Mitchell P, Rochtchina E et al (2003) Prevalence and associations of dry eye syndrome in an older population: the Blue Mountains Eye Study. Clin Experiment Ophthalmol 31:229–232

Damato BE, Allan D, Murray SB, Lee WR (1984) Senile atrophy of the human lacrimal gland: the contribution of chronic inflammatory disease. Br J Ophthalmol 68:674–680

Danjo Y, Lee M, Horimoto K, Hamano T (1994) Ocular surface damage and tear lactoferrin in dry eye syndrome. Acta Ophthalmol 72:433–437

Debbasch C, Pisella PJ, Rat P et al (2000) Evaluation of free radical production by conjunctival impression cytology of patients treated with long-term antiglaucoma drugs or of contact lens wearers. J Fr Ophtalmol 23:239–244

Dogru M, Ishida K, Matsumoto Y et al (2006) Strip meniscometry: a new and simple method of tear meniscus evaluation. Invest Ophthalmol Vis Sci 47:1895–1901

Dogru M, Matsumoto Y, Yamamoto Y, Goto E, Saiki M et al (2007) Lactoferrin in Sjogren's syndrome. Ophthalmology 114:2366–2367

Draper CE, Adeghate E, Lawrence PA, Pallot DJ, Garner A, Singh J (1998) Age-related changes in morphology and secretory responses of male rat lacrimal gland. J Auton Nerv Syst 69:173–183

Frisard M, Ravussin E (2006) Energy metabolism and oxidative stress: impact on the metabolic syndrome and the aging process. Endocrine 29:27–32

Fujihara T, Murakami T, Fujita H et al (2001) Improvement of corneal barrier function by the P2S(2) agonist INS365 in a rat dry eye model. Invest Ophthalmol Vis Sci 42:96–100

Fujihara T, Murakami T, Nagano T et al (2002) INS365 suppresses loss of corneal epithelial integrity by secretion of mucin-like glycoprotein in a rabbit short-term dry eye model. J Ocul Pharmacol Ther 18:363–370

Goto E, Dogru M, Kojima T, Tsubota K (2003) Computer-synthesis of an interference color chart of human tear lipid layer, by a colorimetric approach. Invest Ophthalmol Vis Sci 44:4693–4697

Goto E, Ishida R, Kaido M (2006) Optical aberrations and visual disturbances associated with dry eye. Ocul Surf 4:207–213. Review

Gritz DC, Montes C, Atalla LR, Wu GS, Sevanian A, Rao NA (1991) Histochemical localization of superoxide production in experimental autoimmune uveitis. Curr Eye Res 10:927–931

Guarente L (2008) Mitochondria—a nexus for aging, calorie restriction, and sirtuins? Cell 132:171–176

Haegerstrom-Portnoy G, Schneck ME, Brabyn JA (1999) Seeing into old age: vision function beyond acuity. Optom Vis Sci 76:141–158

Harman D (1956) Aging: a theory based on free radical and radiation chemistry. J Gerontol 11:298–300

Heilbronn LK, de Jonge L, Frisard MI et al (2006) Effect of 6-month calorie restriction on biomarkers of longevity, metabolic adaptation, and oxidative stress in overweight individuals: a randomized controlled trial. JAMA 295:1539–1548

Higuchi A, Takahashi K, Hirashima M, Kawakita T, Tsubota K (2010) Selenoprotein P controls oxidative stress in cornea. PLoS One 5(3):e9911

Horwath J, Schmut O (2000) The influence of environmental factors on the development of dry eye. Contactologia 22:21–29

Horwath-Winter J, Schmut O, Haller-Schober EM, Gruber A, Rieger G (2005) Iodide iontophoresis as a treatment for dry eye syndrome. Br J Ophthalmol 89:40–44

Ibrahim OMA, Dogru M, Ward SK, Matsumoto Y, Wakamatsu T, Ishida K, Tsuyama A, Kojima T, Shimazaki J, Tsubota K (2011) The efficacy, sensitivity, and specificity of strip meniscometry in conjunction with tear function tests in the assessment of tear meniscus. Invest Ophthalmol Vis Sci 52:2194–2198

Imamura Y, Noda S, Hashizume K, Shinoda K, Yamaguchi M, Uchiyama S et al (2006) Drusen, choroidal neovascularization, and retinal pigment epithelium dysfunction in SOD1-deficient mice: a model of age-related macular degeneration. Proc Natl Acad Sci U S A 103:11282–11287

Ishida R, Kojima T, Dogru M, Kaido M, Matsumoto Y, Tanaka M, Goto E, Tsubota K (2005) The application of a new continuous functional visual acuity measurement system in dry eye syndromes. Am J Ophthalmol 139:253–258

Jensen OL, Gluud BS, Birgens HS (1986) The concentration of lactoferrin in tears of normals and of diabetics. Acta Ophthalmol (Copenh) 64:83–87

Kaido M, Matsumoto Y, Shigeno Y, Ishida R, Dogru M, Tsubota K (2011) Corneal fluorescein staining correlates with visual function in dry eye patients. Invest Ophthalmol Vis Sci 52:9516–9522

Kaido M, Ishida R, Dogru M, Tsubota K (2012a) Visual function changes after punctal occlusion with the treatment of short BUT type of dry eye. Cornea 31:1009–1013

Kaido M, Yamada M, Sotozono C, Kinoshita S, Shimazaki J, Tagawa Y, Hara Y, Chikama T, Tsubota K (2012b) The relation between visual performance and clinical ocular manifestations in Stevens-Johnson syndrome. Am J Ophthalmol 154:499–511

Kaido M, Uchino M, Kojima T, Dogru M, Tsubota K (2013) Effects of diquafosol tetrasodium administration on visual function in short break-up time dry eye. J Ocul Pharmacol Ther 29(6):595–603

Kamoi M, Ogawa Y, Nakamura S, Dogru M, Nagai T et al (2012) Accumulation of secretory vesicles in the lacrimal gland epithelia is related to non-sjogren's type dry eye in visual display terminal users. PLoS One 7(9): e43688

Kanyshkova TG, Buneva VN, Nevinsky GA (2001) Lactoferrin and its biological functions. Biochemistry (Mosc) 66:1–7

Kawashima M, Kawakita T, Okada N, Ogawa Y, Murat D, Nakamura S, Nakashima H, Shimmura S, Shinmura K, Tsubota K (2010) Calorie restriction: a new therapeutic intervention for age-related dry eye disease in rats. Biochem Biophys Res Commun 397(4):724–728

Kawashima M, Kawakita T, Inaba T, Okada N, Ito M, Shimmura S, Watanabe M, Shinmura K, Tsubota K (2012) Dietary lactoferrin alleviates age-related lacrimal gland dysfunction in mice. PLoS One 7(3):e33148

Koh S, Maeda N, Hori Y, Inoue T, Watanabe H, Hirohara Y, Mihashi T, Fujikado T, Tano Y (2008) Effects of suppression of blinking on quality of vision in borderline cases of evaporative dry eye. Cornea 27:275–278

Kojima T, Ibrahim OM, Wakamatsu T, Tsuyama A, Ogawa J et al (2011) The impact of contact lens wear and visual display terminal work on ocular surface and tear functions in office workers. Am J Ophthalmol 152:933–940

Kunlin J (2010) Modern biological theories of aging. Aging Dis 1:72–74

Lemp MA, Bron AJ, Baudouinm C et al (2011) Tear osmolarity in the diagnosis and management of dry eye disease. Am J Ophthalmol 151:792–798

Legrand D, Elass E, Carpentier M, Mazurier J (2005) Lactoferrin: a modulator of immune and inflammatory responses. Cell Mol Life Sci 62:2549–2559

Lemp MA, Foulks GN (2007) Definition and Classification of Dry Eye. Report of the Diagnosis and Classification Subcommittee of the Dry Eye Workshop (DEWS). Ocul Surf 5(2):75–92

Lemp MA, Foulks GN, Pepose JS (2013) Evaluation of tear osmolarity in non-Sjögren and Sjögren syndrome dry eye patients with the TearLab system. Cornea 32:379–381

Lin PY, Tsai SY, Cheng CY et al (2003) Prevalence of dry eye among an elderly Chinese population in Taiwan: the Shihpai Eye Study. Ophthalmology 110:1096–1101

Longo VD, Kennedy BK (2006) Sirtuins in aging and age-related disease. Cell 126:257–268

Masoro EJ (2000) Caloric restriction and aging: an update. Exp Gerontol 35:299–305

Matsuzawa Y (2006) Therapy insight: adipocytokines in metabolic syndrome and related cardiovascular disease. Nat Clin Pract Cardiovasc Med 3:35–42

McGill JI, Liakos GM, Goulding N, Seal DV (1984) Normal tear protein profiles and age-related changes. Br J Ophthalmol 68:316–320

Miljanović B, Trivedi KA, Dana MR, Gilbard JP, Buring JE, Schaumberg DA (2005) Relation between dietary n-3 and n-6 fatty acids and clinically diagnosed dry eye syndrome in women. Am J Clin Nutr 82: 887–893

Montes-Mico R, Caliz A, Alio JL (2004) Changes in ocular aberrations after instillation of artificial tears in dry-eye patients. J Cataract Refract Surg 30:1649–1652

Moss SE, Klein R, Klein BE (2000) Prevalence of and risk factors for dry eye syndrome. Arch Ophthalmol 118:1264–1268

Nakamura S, Shibuya M, Nakashima H, Hisamura R, Masuda N, Imagawa T et al (2007) Involvement of oxidative stress on corneal epithelial alterations in a blink suppressed dry eye. Invest Ophthalmol Vis Sci 48:1552–1558

Nakamura S, Kinoshita S, Yokoi N, Ogawa Y, Shibuya M et al (2010) Lacrimal hypofunction as a new mechanism of dry eye in visual display terminal users. PLoS One 5:e11119

Nichols JJ, Sinnott LT (2006) Tear film, contact lens, and patient-related factors associated with contact lens-related dry eye. Invest Ophthalmol Vis Sci 47: 1319–1328

Niesman MR, Johnson KA, Penn JS (1997) Therapeutic effect of liposomal superoxide dismutase in an animal model of retinopathy of prematurity. Neurochem Res 22:597–605

Obata H, Yamamoto S, Horiuchi H, Machinami R (1995) Histopathologic study of human lacrimal gland. Statistical analysis with special reference to aging. Ophthalmology 102:678–686

Paradies G, Petrosillo G, Paradies V, Ruggiero FM (2010) Oxidative stress, mitochondrial bioenergetics and cardiolipin in aging. Free Radic Biol Med 48:1286–1295

Pearson KJ, Baur JA, Lewis KN et al (2008) Resveratrol delays age-related deterioration and mimics transcriptional aspects of dietary restriction without extending life span. Cell Metab 8:157–168

Ridder WH 3rd, Tomlinson A, Paugh J (2005) Effect of artificial tears on visual performance in subjects with dry eye. Optom Vis Sci 82:835–842

Ridder WH 3rd, Tomlinson A, Huang JF, Li J (2011) Impaired visual performance in patients with dry eye. Ocul Surf 9:42–55

Ríos JD, Horikawa Y, Chen LL, Kublin CL, Hodges RR, Dartt DA, Zoukhri D (2005) Age-dependent alterations in mouse exorbital lacrimal gland structure, innervation and secretory response. Exp Eye Res 80:477–491

Rios JD, Shatos M, Urachima H, Tran H, Dartt DA (2006) OPC-12759 increases proliferation of cultured rat conjunctival goblet cells. Cornea 25:573–581

Rios JD, Shatos MA, Urashima H, Dartt DA (2008) Effect of OPC-12759 on EGF receptor activation, p44/p42 MAPK activity, and secretion in conjunctival goblet cells. Exp Eye Res 86:629–636

Schaumberg DA, Sullivan DA, Buring JE, Dana MR (2003) Prevalence of dry eye syndrome among US women. Am J Ophthalmol 136:318–326

Schaumberg DA, Dana R, Buring JE, Sullivan DA (2009) Prevalence of dry eye disease among US men: estimates from the Physicians' Health Studies. Arch Ophthalmol 127:763–768

Schein OD, Muñoz B, Tielsch JM et al (1997) Prevalence of dry eye among the elderly. Am J Ophthalmol 124:723–728

Smith JA, Albeitz J, Begley C et al (2007) The epidemiology of dry eye disease: report of the epidemiology subcommittee of the international dry eye workshop. Ocul Surf 5:75.92

Spector A (1995) Oxidative stress-induced cataract: mechanism of action. FASEB J 9:1173–1182

Spindler SR (2001) Calorie restriction enhances the expression of key metabolic enzymes associated with protein renewal during aging. Ann N Y Acad Sci 928:296–304

Sullivan DA, Hann LE, Yee L, Allansmith MR (1990) Age- and gender-related influence on the lacrimal gland and tears. Acta Ophthalmol (Copenh) 68:188–194

Sullivan BD, Whitmer D, Nichols KK et al (2010) An objective approach to dry eye disease severity. Invest Ophthalmol Vis Sci 51:6125–6130

Sullivan BD, Crews LA, Sonmez B et al (2012) Clinical utility of objective tests for dry eye disease: variability over time and implications for clinical trials and disease management. Cornea 31:1000–1001

Takaoka-Shichijo Y, Nakamura M (2011) Stimulatory effect of diquafosol tetrasodium on the expression of membrane-binding mucin genes in cultured human corneal epithelial cells. J Eye 28:425–429

Toda I, Fumishima H, Tsubota K (1993) Ocular fatigue is a major symptom of dry eye. Acta Ophthalmol 71:347–352

Toda I, Shimazaki J, Tsubota K (1995) Dry eye with only decreased tear break-up time is sometimes associated with allergic conjunctivitis. Ophthalmology 102:302–309

Tong L, Waduthantri S, Wong TY et al (2010) Impact of symptomatic dry eye on vision related daily activities: the Singapore Malay Eye study. Eye (Lond) 24:1486–1491

Tsubota K, Nakamori K (1993) Dry eye and video display terminals. N Engl J Med 25:584

Tsubota K, Nakamori K (1995) Effects of ocular surface area and blink rate on tear dynamics. Arch Ophthalmol 113:155–158

Tsubota K, Toda I, Nakamori K (1996) Poor illumination, VDTs, and desiccated eyes. Lancet 347:768–769

Uchida M, Tabusa F, Komatsu M et al (1985) Studies on 2(IH)-quinolinone derivatives as gastric antiulcer active agents. 2-(4-Chlorobenzoylamino)-3-[2(IH)-quinolinon-4-yl]propionic acid and related compounds. Chem Pharm Bull (Tokyo) 33:3775–3786

Uchino M, Dogru M, Yagi Y, Goto E, Tomita M, Kon T, Saiki M, Matsumoto Y, Uchino Y, Yokoi N, Kinoshita S, Tsubota K (2006) The features of dry eye disease in a Japanese elderly population. Optom Vis Sci 83:797–802

Urashima H, Okamoto T, Takeji Y, Shinohara H, Fujisawa S (2004) Rebamipide increases the amount of mucin-like substances on the conjunctiva and cornea in the N-acetylcysteine-treated in vivo model. Cornea 23:613–619

Valentine JS, Doucette PA, Zittin Potter S (2005) Copper-zinc superoxide dismutase and amyotrophic lateral sclerosis. Annu Rev Biochem 74:563–593

Versura P, Profazio V, Cellini M et al (1999) Eye discomfort and air pollution. Ophthalmologica 213:103–109

Viso E, Rodriguez-Ares MT, Gude F (2009) Prevalence of and associated factors for dry eye in a Spanish adult population (the Salnes Eye Study). Ophthalmic Epidemiol 16:15–21

Williams RM, Singh J, Sharkey KA (1994) Innervation and mast cells of the rat exorbital lacrimal gland: the effects of age. J Auton Nerv Syst 47:95–108

Walker PM, Lone KJ, Ousler GW 3rd, Abelson MB (2010) Diurnal variation of visual function and the signs and symptoms of dry eye. Cornea 29:607–612

Watanabe H (2002) Significance of mucin on the ocular surface. Cornea 21:17–22

Zimniak P (2008) Detoxification reactions: relevance to aging. Ageing Res Rev 7:281–300

Jennifer P. Craig, Colin Chan, Marcella Salomão,
Fernando Faria Correia, Isaac Ramos,
Renato Ambrósio Jr , Victor L. Caparas,
Minako Kaido, and Kazuo Tsubota

8.1 MGD Case Report

Jennifer P. Craig

8.1.1 Background

A 31-year-old female (RM), diagnosed with moderate dry eye 6 months previously by her ophthalmologist, was referred to the Ocular Surface Laboratory (OSL) for an opinion on optimal management of her condition. Experiencing constant burning and grittiness symptoms, and with relief only when sleeping, RM found her quality of life had deteriorated and her ability to function at work for a full day, without severely curtailing her activities, was impaired. Computer work was described as difficult and prolonged

J.P. Craig, PhD, MCOptom (✉)
Department of Ophthalmology, New Zealand
National Eye Centre, The University of Auckland,
Auckland, New Zealand
e-mail: jp.craig@auckland.ac.nz

C. Chan, MBBS (Hons) FRANZCO
Vision Eye Institute, School of Optometry and Vision
Science, University of New South Wales,
270 Victoria Ave, Chatswood, Sydney,
NSW 2067, Australia
e-mail: colin.chan@visioneyeinstitute.com.au

M. Salomão, MD
Instituto de Olhos Renato Ambrósio,
Rio de Janeiro, Brazil

Rio de Janeiro Corneal Tomography and
Biomechanics Study Group, Rio de Janeiro, Brazil

Department of Ophthalmology, Federal University of
Sao Paulo, Sao Paulo, Brazil

F.F. Correia, MD
Instituto de Olhos Renato Ambrósio,
Rio de Janeiro, Brazil

Rio de Janeiro Corneal Tomography and
Biomechanics Study Group, Rio de Janeiro, Brazil

Department of Ophthalmology, University of Porto,
Porto, Portugal

I. Ramos, MD
Instituto de Olhos Renato Ambrósio,
Rio de Janeiro, Brazil

Rio de Janeiro Corneal Tomography and
Biomechanics Study Group, Rio de Janeiro, Brazil

Cataract and Refractive Surgery, Hospital de Olhos
Santa Luzia, Gruta de Lourdes,
Maceió, Alagoas, Brazil

R. Ambrósio Jr, MD, PhD
Rio de Janeiro Corneal Tomography and
Biomechanics Study Group, Rio de Janeiro, Brazil

Department of Ophthalmology, Federal University
of Sao Paulo, Sao Paulo, Brazil

Instituto de Olhos Renato Ambrósio, VisareRIO
Refracta Personal Laser, Rio de Janeiro, Brazil

V.L. Caparas, MD, MPH
Department of Ophthalmology, The Medical City,
Medical Arts Tower, Suite 1912, Ortigas Avenue,
Pasig City, Metro Manila 1600, Philippines
e-mail: victor.caparas@gmail.com

M. Kaido, MD, PhD • K. Tsubota, MD
Department of Ophthalmology,
Keio University School of Medicine,
Shinjuku-ku, Tokyo, Japan

C. Chan (ed.), *Dry Eye: A Practical Approach*, Essentials in Ophthalmology,
DOI 10.1007/978-3-662-44106-0_8, © Springer-Verlag Berlin Heidelberg 2015

screen use, impossible. Any requirement to attend meetings in air-conditioned rooms caused significant concern and she would often have to leave early on account of debilitating symptoms. In the 6 months prior to referral to the OSL, RM had trialled an extensive range of lubricant eye drops, had been prescribed a course of doxycycline (50 mg daily for 12 weeks) and had been prescribed intermittent courses of topical steroids (prednisolone acetate 0.12 % ophthalmic emulsion by day and dexamethasone 0.1 % ointment at night) and topical antibiotics (chloramphenicol). RM reported that these products did not appear to have made any difference to the symptoms she experienced and, indeed in some cases, had exacerbated her symptoms. On referral, RM was performing twice daily lid hygiene and her aqueous deficiency was being managed, as instructed by her ophthalmologist, with punctal occlusion (Sharpoint Silicone Plugs, InterMed Medical Ltd., NZ), twice daily topical cyclosporin emulsion (0.2 %) (Optimis Pharmacy, Penrose, Auckland, NZ) and non-preserved topical lubricants, as required (Systane Ultra, Alcon and LacriLube ointment, Allergan, at night).

8.1.2 Evaluation

At her first OSL visit, RM's eyes were visibly inflamed, and, on detailed questioning, she reported that in addition to ocular irritation symptoms, she experienced significant oral dryness symptoms and an apparent inability to reflex tear under usual circumstances. A comprehensive battery of tests evaluating ocular surface health and function was thus performed in an attempt to ascertain the cause of RM's distressing discomfort.

Subjective assessment of established symptoms and risk factors for dry eye, as well as recently experienced symptoms, was undertaken with the McMonnies Dry Eye Questionnaire and the OSDI (Ocular Surface Disease Index), respectively (Nichols et al. 2004; Schiffman et al. 2000). High scoring on both dry eye questionnaires was indicative of severe dry eye symptoms. Non-invasive objective testing demonstrated the presence of a tear meniscus with some irregularity along the length of the lid margin and a modest central tear meniscus height of 0.1 mm. Phenol red thread (PRT) and non-anaesthetised Schirmer testing also showed reduced lacrimal gland function, implicating aqueous deficiency as a contributor to the dry eye status in this case.

Evaporative dry eye was also confirmed through evaluations of the tear lipid layer by interferometry (Keeler Tearscope Plus™). This highlighted an intermittently visible lipid layer that would be classified as an absent/open meshwork pattern (Guillon and Guillon 1993), equivalent to a lipid grade of 0/1. Correspondingly high tear evaporation rates (Delfin Vapometer, Finland) and tear osmolarity (TearLab, USA) and low non-invasive break-up times (Keeler Tearscope Plus™, UK) were recorded in both eyes. Slit lamp examination of the eyelid margins revealed signs typical of MGD with lid margin thickening, mild telangiectasia and marked keratinisation along the lid margin and over the orifices of the meibomian glands, particularly in the lower eyelids. Mild crusting of the eyelashes, characteristic of staphylococcal blepharitis, was also observed, predominantly on the upper eyelids.

Infrared meibography (SDZ Electronics, Auckland, NZ) confirmed limited meibomian gland drop out, with mild irregularity of gland morphology in the upper eyelid and evidence of truncation and moderate inspissation of the inferior glands (Fig. 8.1). Manual gland expression with the aid of a posteriorly placed Mastrota paddle (OcuSoft, USA) yielded minimal discharge from the glands.

RM's corneal integrity appeared relatively unaffected by her tear film condition, as confirmed by fluorescein and lissamine green staining. However, there was moderate conjunctival staining with lissamine green in the inter-palpebral zone, particularly nasally, indicating the presence of dead or devitalised cells, or cells devoid of surface glyco-calyx, rendering

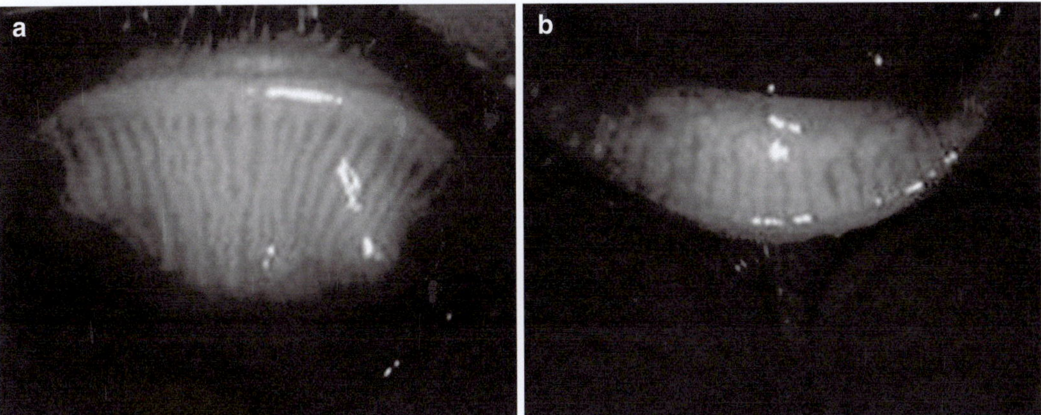

Fig. 8.1 (**a**) Upper lid meibography. (**b**) Lower lid meibography

them hydrophobic in nature (Hamrah et al. 2011).

8.1.3 Management

A staged approach to dry eye management was implemented, in recognition of the need to adopt a multifaceted approach to ameliorating symptoms arising from a multifactorial condition. The breadth of tear film and ocular surface features, found to be compromised in this patient, indicated a diagnosis of combined aqueous deficiency and evaporative dry eye. The approaches by which these aspects were addressed are described in turn.

8.1.3.1 Aqueous Deficiency
The combination of punctal occlusion, topical cyclosporin (0.2 %) and topical lubricants prescribed by RM's ophthalmologist was, at the time of referral, well tolerated by the patient and was proving sufficient to maintain a modest volume tear meniscus. The management plan for this aspect was not altered, therefore, particularly in light of reported sensitivities to a number of eye products previously, including a lipid/aqueous combination product. The account of symptoms of dry mouth, as well as dry eye, however, suggested the possibility of underlying systemic disease and prompted serological evaluation, to test for auto-antibodies pertinent to Sjögren's syndrome. These included

rheumatoid factor (RF), anti-nuclear antibodies (ANA), anti-SS-A/Ro and anti-SS-B/La. While RM tested sero-negative to these antibodies, at this time, it was recognised that unequivocally discounting a diagnosis of Sjögren's syndrome was not justified. Antibodies against SSA/Ro are identified in only around 50 % of patients with Sjögren's syndrome, while antibodies against SSB/La are found in even fewer, around 30 % of patients with Sjögren's syndrome (Huo et al. 2010). Fractionally borderline results for some of the antibodies in RM's case indicated that repeat evaluation in the future might be warranted.

8.1.3.2 Evaporative Dry Eye
With serological testing underway, the next step following referral to the Ocular Surface Laboratory was to direct treatment towards RM's meibomian gland dysfunction and its sequelae. On presentation, RM had been performing regular, twice-daily lid cleansing with a commercial lid preparation, followed by 10-min, warm compress treatments with a microwave-heated wheat bag, according to the advice of her ophthalmologist. Subjectively RM reported modest symptomatic relief from these treatments. After confirming appropriate lid cleansing, warming and expression techniques were being performed by RM; further advice was provided with regard to environmental exposure. The modification to the environment recommended in this case involved,

not only minimising exposure to low relative humidity environments created by air conditioning and exposure to high air flow environments but also avoiding exposure to airborne chemicals with the potential to destabilise the tear film. RM described having worked in a building situated adjacent to a vehicle paint-spraying site where exposure to noxious fumes from paint and associated chemicals was a regular occurrence. Paint thinner, for example, is primarily a mixture of aliphatic hydrocarbons, the vapours of which are recognised to induce conjunctival and corneal irritation and inflammation (Bulbulia et al. 1995). Goggles that create a seal around the skin protect the local environment which can help with maintaining higher levels of moisture around the exposed ocular surface (Alex et al. 2013; Korb and Blackie 2013b) and can also reduce exposure to airborne irritants. Spectacles with foam inserts perform a similar function, with superior cosmetic acceptability, and therefore were recommended in this instance (http://www.7eye.com/) and resulted in symptomatic improvement. Interestingly, in this case, the patient's subsequent decision to change her job made a further noticeable difference to the severity of her ocular discomfort symptoms, corroborating the belief that airborne pollutants were a significant factor in exacerbating her dry eye condition.

RM's low-lipid delivery state was deemed to be the result of obstruction of the gland orifices due to significant keratinisation that could be observed extending onto the lid margin surface (Fig. 8.2a). Hyperkeratinisation of the meibomian ductal system is recognised to be a core mechanism in the development of obstructive MGD (Henriquez and Korb 1981; Knop et al. 2011).

The decision was made to debride the lid margin, in an effort to facilitate egress of the meibomian fluid from the inferior glands (Korb and Blackie 2013a). Topical anaesthesia of the eyelid margin with oxybuprocaine 0.4 %, (Bausch & Lomb) was followed by staining with lissamine green (Fig. 8.2b) to highlight the keratinised areas. Utilising the magnification of the slit lamp, the surface of the lid margin was carefully debrided with a golf club spud (Fig. 8.2c), and the excess keratinised material gently removed. The resulting lid margin profile was significantly smoother as seen in Fig. 8.2d, and the number of glands yielding secretion markedly increased. To date, this improvement has been maintained for over 8 months, post-treatment.

Debridement was thus successful in facilitating meibum outflow from the glands, but, somewhat disappointingly, it was observed that the lipid layer created, following debridement, was of poor quality and the tear film lacked stability,

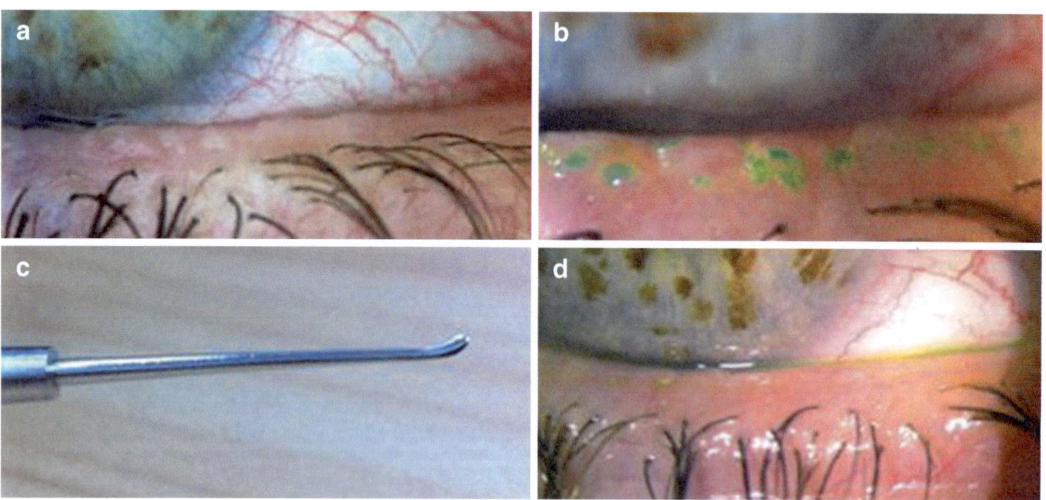

Fig. 8.2 (**a**) Lower lid hyperkeratinisation; (**b**) hyperkeratinisation stained with lissamine green; (**c**) golf club spatula for debridement; (**d**) lid quality post-debridement

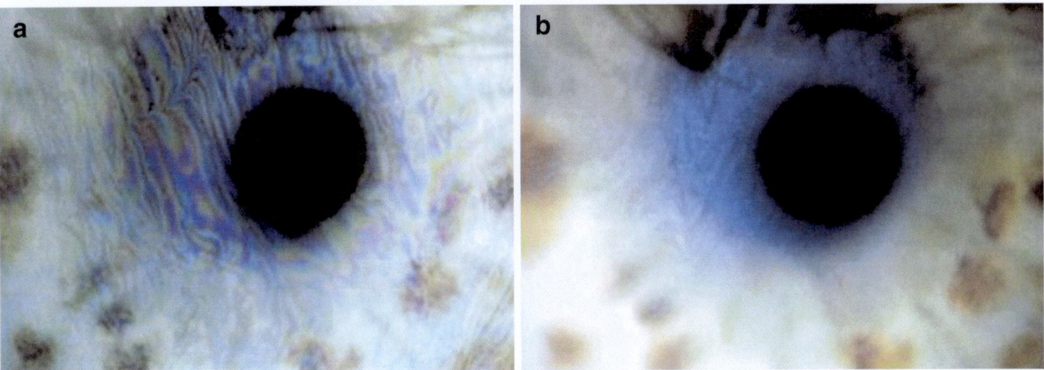

Fig. 8.3 (**a**) Non-confluent lipid cover pre-omega-3 therapy, grade 0. (**b**) Confluent lipid layer post-omega-3 therapy, grade 2/3

as indicated by a non-invasive break-up time of less than 4 s. The abnormal coloured fringes that were visible (Fig. 8.3a) suggested the presence of lipid globules amidst areas of little or no lipid cover (Guillon and Guillon 1993). Without confluence, such a layer is believed incapable of performing its required function of inhibiting tear evaporation (Craig and Tomlinson 1997).

A means of modifying the lipid quality was therefore sought. Low-dose doxycycline taken over an extended period (e.g. 50 mg daily for 2–3 months) is a well-established therapy for improving gland function in MGD (Sobolewska et al. 2014) and was thus considered as a potential therapy. Reflecting their anti-inflammatory rather than anti-bacterial properties, low-dose tetracyclines improve lipid quality on account of their ability to suppress the production of the bacterial lipases which otherwise serve to destabilise the tear film in MGD (Dougherty et al. 1991). Our patient, however, had not tolerated doxycycline well during a previously prescribed course and was reluctant to commence further doxycycline treatment. It was elected therefore to adopt a more natural approach to lipid layer alteration, through diet. Essential fatty acid supplementation has recognised anti-inflammatory effects throughout the body, due competitive inhibition, between the omega-3 fatty acid, eicosapentaenoic acid, and omega-6 fatty acid, arachidonic acid, to synthesise mediators with anti-inflammatory properties over potentially harmful inflammatory mediators (James et al. 2000). Mounting

evidence suggests positive effects in MGD from dietary supplementation with omega-3 fatty acids, with a recent randomised, placebo-controlled, trial describing improvements in symptomatology as well as in clinical signs such as lid margin inflammation, meibomian gland expression, tear film stability and tear production (Olenik et al. 2013).

Such improvements were, indeed, realised following a conscious effort by RM to increase her omega-3 intake, both naturally from the regular consumption of smoked salmon and in the form of a nutritional supplement. After an 8-week period, her non-invasive break-up time was noted to have increased by around 3.5 s, in tandem with an improvement in her lipid layer quality to a marmoreal/wave combination pattern (thickness around 60–80 nm), implying presence of a confluent lipid layer (Fig. 8.3b) (Guillon and Guillon 1993). Tear evaporation rate was correspondingly decreased.

A concurrent reduction in bulbar conjunctival hyperaemia (Fig. 8.4) and symptoms was also noted, following the lid margin debridement and the described change in diet.

Following the dietary changes, RM's tear film and ocular surface condition was observed to stabilise and symptoms were described as tolerable, although not fully ameliorated. With the hope of achieving further symptomatic relief, RM thus opted to engage in an opportunity to trial treatment with the E > Eye Intense Pulsed Light (IPL) device for MGD within the

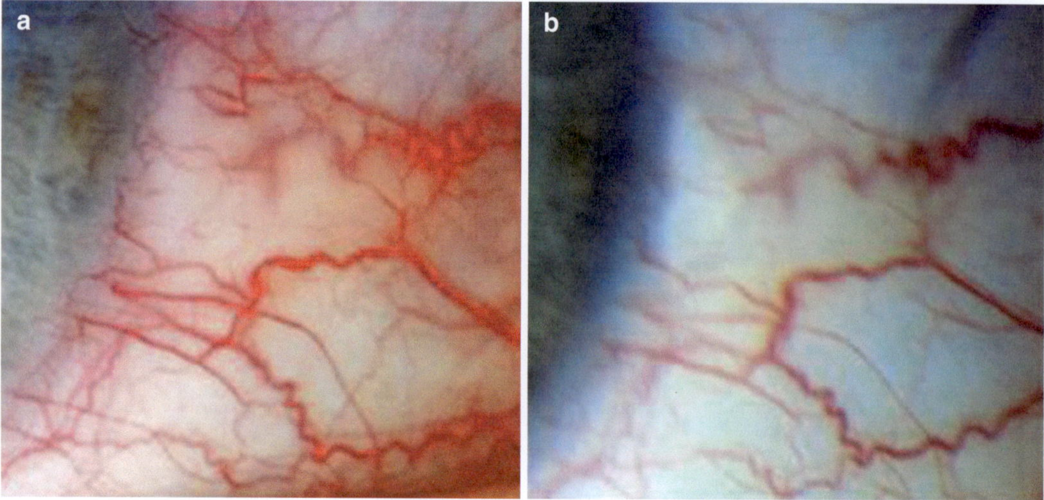

Fig. 8.4 Bulbar hyperaemia pre- (**a**) and post (**b**)-lid margin debridement and omega-3 treatment

Ocular Surface Laboratory. The potential benefits of IPL technology, as an MGD therapy, were discovered during cosmetic IPL skin treatments for patients with acne rosacea, where it was noted that individuals with associated ocular rosacea experienced concurrent improvements in their dry eye condition following IPL treatment on the upper cheek area of the face (Mark et al. 2003). Toyos in the United States is a firm proponent of IPL for MGD on the basis of his personal clinical findings (Toyos et al. 2005). However, the reports of these open-label treatments require validation with randomised, placebo-controlled trials to confirm the true benefit. Certainly, from an anecdotal perspective, patient RM has experienced further improvement in meibomian gland function since commencing monthly IPL treatments, with both immediate and sustained increases in lipid layer quality. She currently exhibits an amorphous/normal coloured fringe pattern, corresponding to lipid grade 4/5 (Fig. 8.5), and this has been associated with a reduction in ocular discomfort symptoms.

At the present time, RM is enjoying significantly reduced irritation symptoms, in comparison to those on presentation, and is delighted with the reduction in her red eye appearance. Her quality of life has improved significantly, such that she can now work a full day without marked

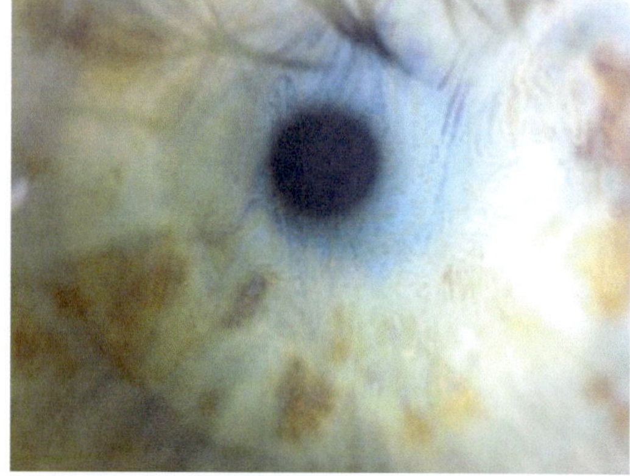

Fig. 8.5 Confluent lipid layer, post-IPL, grade 4/5

restrictions on her activities. She continues with cyclosporin therapy, punctal occlusion and artificial lubricants as required, supplemented with ointment at night. Due to hypertrophy of the punctum secondary to silicone punctal plugs, which was causing intermittent mechanical irritation, a more permanent solution to punctal occlusion has recently been sought with cautery to replace the silicone plugs. Lid hygiene, warm compress therapy and manual expression form part of a daily routine for RM. These ongoing strategies, applied in conjunction with lid margin debridement, dietary regulation and monthly IPL treatments, have, in the words of this individual, 'given her back her life'.

8.2 Dry Eye Case Report 1

Colin Chan

A 56-year-old self-employed lady was referred by her optometrist with a several year history of dry eye and contact lens tolerance issues. Previous treatments had included TheraTears drops, TheraTears flaxseed and fish oil supplement, Zaditen and warm compresses, all of which had provided some relief. Serology testing was negative for Sjögren's syndrome. She ultimately wanted to consider a refractive lens exchange because of her contact lens issues and her unsuitability for laser given her underlying dry eye condition.

Initial slit lamp findings were mild sub-tarsal papillary changes and limbal injection in both eyes. There was significant lid margin disease and insippation of the meibomian glands; tear BUT was 3 s in both eyes. Manifest refraction in the right eye was +2.75/−0.25×125 giving 6/7.5 and in the left was +2.75/−0.50×180 yielding 6/7.5. Corneal topography showed regular with the rule astigmatism in both eyes. A diagnosis of dry eye secondary to meibomian gland dysfunction and contact lens keratoconjunctivitis/hypersensitivity was made.

She responded well to an initial pulse of FML tds for 3 weeks. Zaditen tds was reinitiated and the patient asked to continue the omega-3 supplements and warm compresses. TBUT increased to 5 s in both eyes with a decrease in limbal injection.

The patient represented later that year with markedly reduced vision eye and increased irritation especially in the right eye. She stated that things had gotten worse after recent house renovations and a trip to New Zealand. She had worn her contact lenses minimally. Manifest refraction in the right eye was +1.50/−0.75×151 yielding 6/45 only and in the left eye +2.25/−0.25×86 giving 6/18. There was superior haze in her right cornea with overlying punctuate defects and diffuse nummular opacities in her left eye (Figs. 8.6 and 8.7). Topographies showed induced corneal irregular astigmatism (Fig. 8.8a, b).

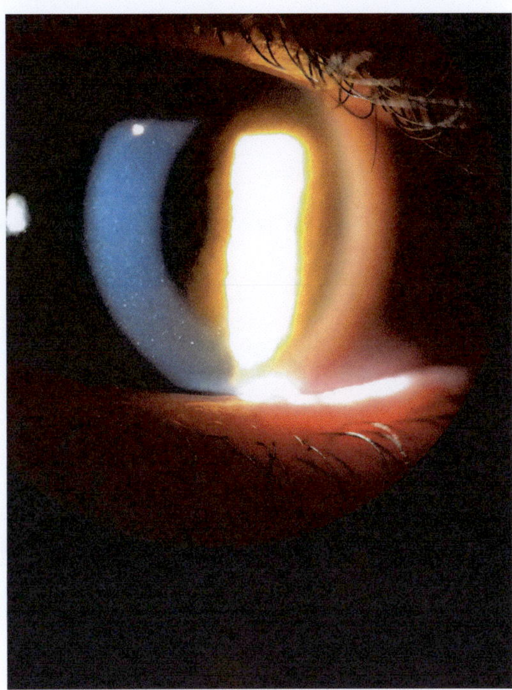

Fig. 8.6 Mild superior corneal haze in right eye

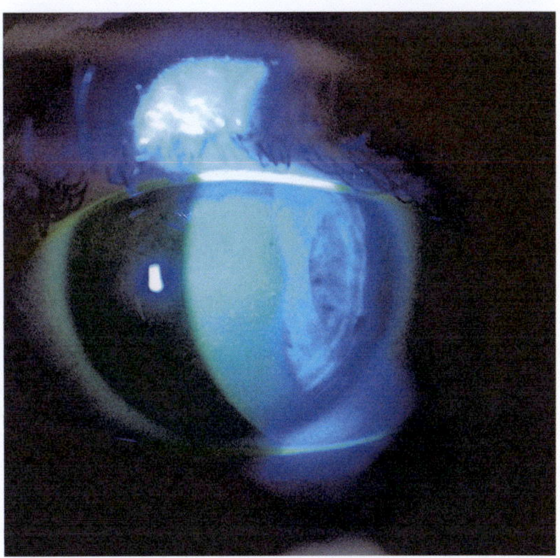

Fig. 8.7 Punctate staining over area of haze typical of nummular or contact lens keratitis

Prednefrine forte tds, Zaditen tds and minocycline 50 mg daily were prescribed. Resolution of the corneal haze and irregular astigmatism took 2 months.

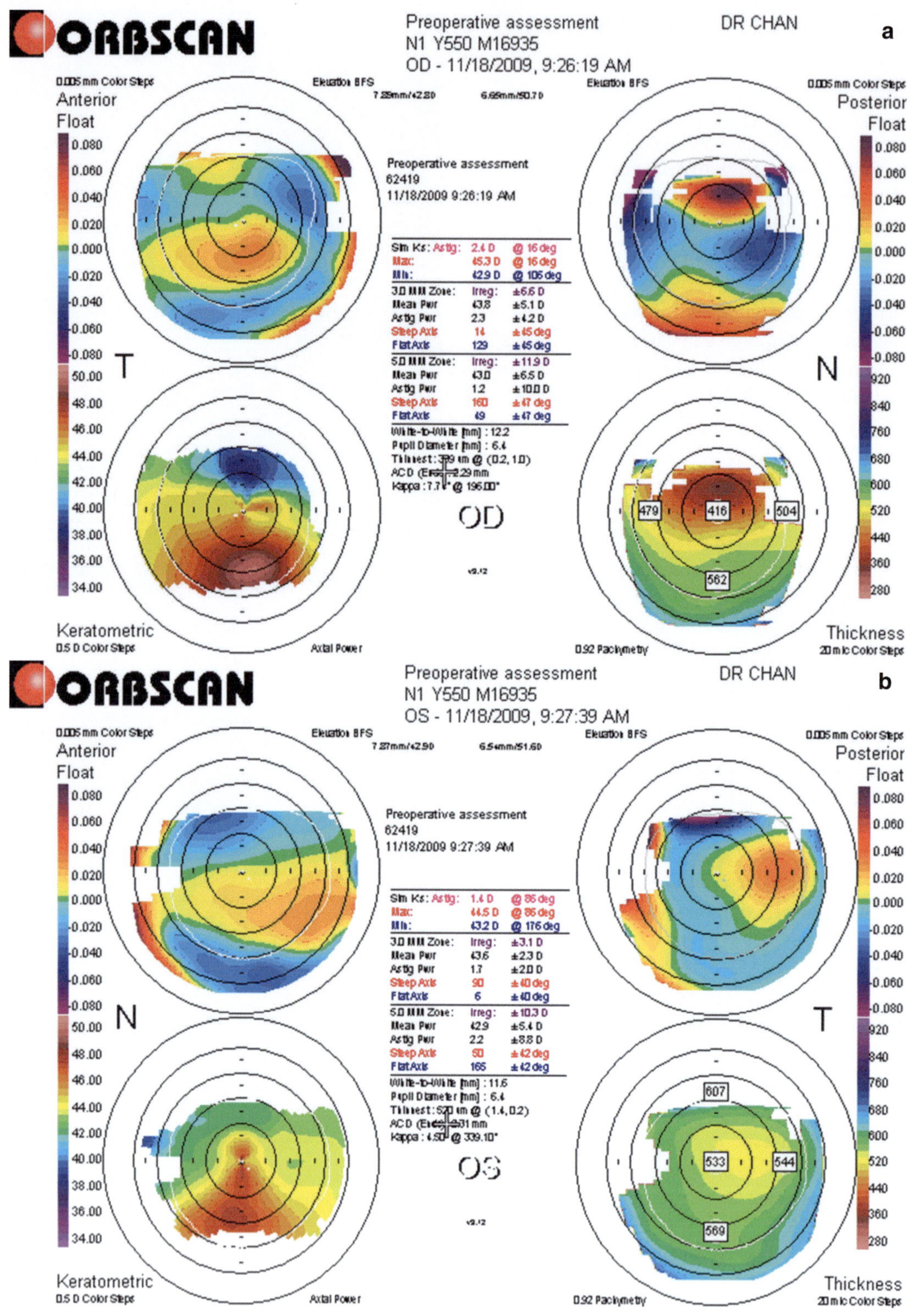

Fig. 8.8 (**a**) Initial topographies on top show regular with the rule astigmatism. (**b**) Topographies below taken at time of keratitis show induced irregular astigmatism resulting in loss of BCVA

8.2.1 Discussion

Dry eye syndrome can increase the likelihood and severity of contact lens kerato-conjunctivitis. This lady had a severe episode of contact lens keratitis with minimal contact lens usage. Loss of BCVA and corneal irregular astigmatism can be permanent if not treated promptly.

Recommended treatment for both severe dry eye syndrome and contact lens keratitis is pulse topical steroids as inflammation is a key component of both these conditions. A dual action anti-histamine and mast cell stabiliser such as Zaditen or Patanol is a useful adjunct both for its anti-allergy properties but also their anti-inflammatory properties. The case also illustrates other treatments that can be used for dry eye including omega-3 supplements and minocycline. Omega-3 supplements have anti-inflammatory properties and change the lipid profile of meibomian gland secretions.

In an older patient a refractive lens exchange is a reasonable alternative to laser especially the presence of dry eye. Dry eye can still be exacerbated by cataract surgery so it is important to optimise the ocular surface prior to surgery. Postoperative measures to minimise dry eye include punctual plugs, omega-3 supplements and a more prolonged topical steroid course.

8.3 Dry Eye Case Report 2

Colin Chan

A 55-year-old lady presented to myself. She presented with a 2-year history of increasingly severe symptoms of dryness, grittiness and a sensation of someone blowing air onto her eye. More recently she had been having pain at nighttime, causing her to wake up several times during the night and put in PolyVisc ointment. She had tried multiple lubricants and seen multiple optometrists and ophthalmologists. She was extremely distressed by her symptoms and could barely function in her job as a teacher. She was otherwise well with no significant medical history. She was experiencing some peri-menopausal

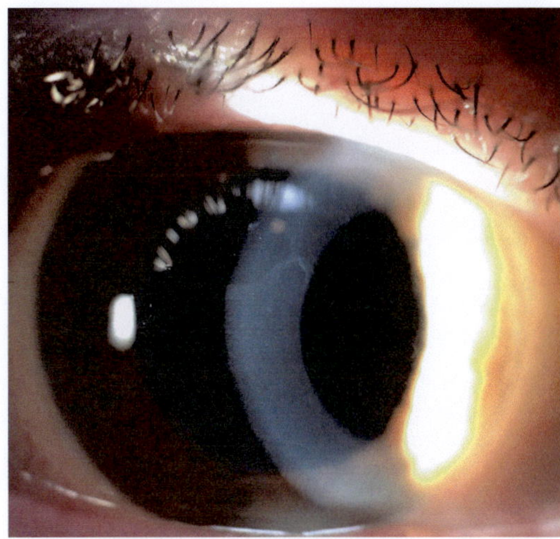

Fig. 8.9 Subepithelial map/fingerprint opacity typical of map dot fingerprint dystrophy

symptoms but was not on hormone replacement therapy. Her Sjögren's serology testing had been negative

Examination findings were:

- Schirmer I score OD 1 mm OS 1 mm
- TBUT OD 1–2 s OS 1–2 s
- Meibomian gland dysfunction +++ OU
- Inferior punctate epithelial erosions OU
- Blepharitis
- Sub-epithelial opacities and negative staining typical of map dot fingerprint dystrophy (Figs. 8.9 and 8.10)

Initially treatment was geared towards improving her meibomian gland dysfunction (MGD) and associated blepharitis with lid scrubs, topical fluorometholone and omega-3 supplements. Doxycycline 100 mg daily was added when there was no subjective improvement in symptoms even though the TBUT improved to 4 s OU. When doxycycline proved ineffective, a trial of punctual plugs was suggested. The patient did not feel the plugs were of any benefit.

I decided to focus instead primarily on the map dot fingerprint dystrophy. I prescribed hypertonic saline 5 % tds, which resulted a definite improvement in symptoms. I then organised serum autologous tears for the patient, and after a few months of using them, the patient became comfortable with no nighttime symptoms in particular.

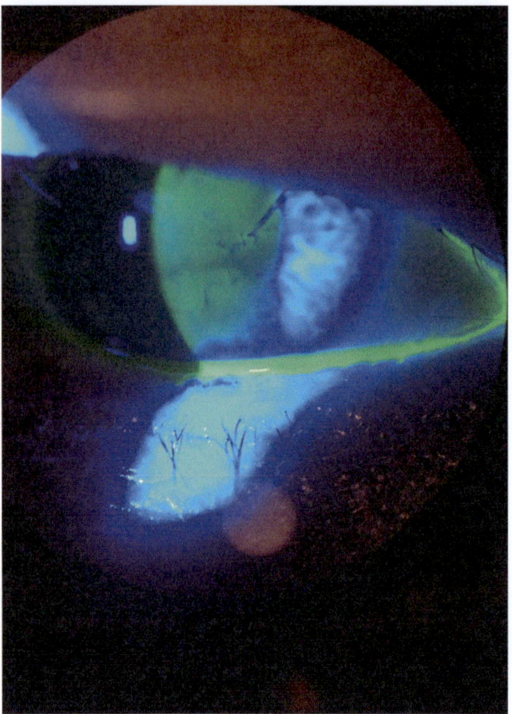

Fig. 8.10 Negative staining with fluorescein indicating epithelial irregularity typical of map dot fingerprint dystrophy

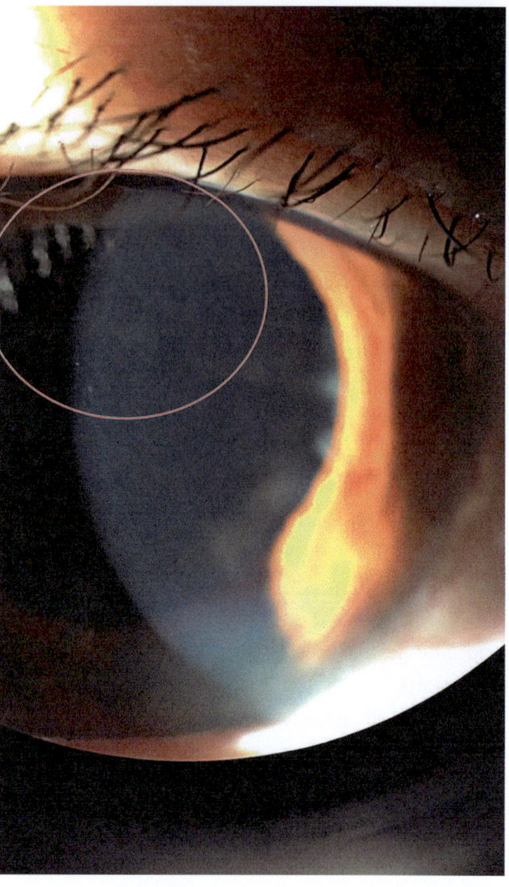

Fig. 8.11 Subepithelial map/fingerprint opacity typical of map dot fingerprint dystrophy

Key Lessons

There are several lessons to be learnt from this case study.

1. Map dot fingerprint (MDF) dystrophy is an often missed diagnosis as it can be asymptomatic initially and the corneal findings quite subtle. It is the most common corneal dystrophy with an incidence of up to 43 %. Only 30 % present with classic symptoms of recurrent erosions. Be suspicious if the patient complains of nighttime dry eye symptoms.

2. MDF dystrophy is more common in females. Clues to diagnosis are:
   - Subtle geographic sub-epithelial white lines typically in the superior cornea – therefore always lift the lid! (Fig. 8.11)
   - Geographic lines of negative staining on fluorescein (Fig. 8.12).
   - Corneal irregularity on topography.

3. MDF dystrophy can mimic dry eye disease. It is also exacerbated by dry eye disease.

4. It can be difficult to determine sometimes if the dry eye or the MDF dystrophy is the primary cause of the patient's symptoms. If the patient's symptoms do not respond to initial dry eye treatment, consider treating the MDF dystrophy specifically with measures such as hypertonic saline or serum autologous tears.

8.4 Dry Eye After LASIK Case Report

Marcella Salomão , Fernando Faria Correia, Isaac Ramos, and Renato Ambrósio Jr

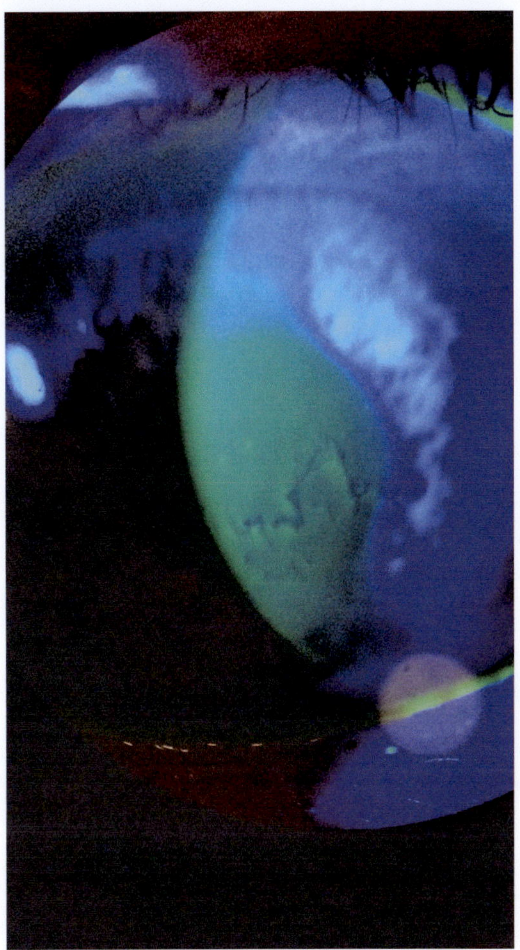

Fig. 8.12 Negative staining with fluorescein indicating epithelial irregularity typical of map dot fingerprint dystrophy

8.4.1 Introduction

Laser in situ keratomileusis (LASIK) is the most commonly performed refractive surgical procedure (Duffey and Leaming 2005). Advances in techniques and instruments have contributed to improve results and minimise complications of LASIK. However, one of the most common problems noted after surgery is LASIK-associated dry eye (Wilson 2001; Ambrósio et al. 2008; Wilson and Ambrósio 2001). This complication is recognised as one of the major causes of patient dissatisfaction and surgeon frustration. LASIK-induced neurotrophic epitheliopathy (LINE), from injure to the nerves during flap formation and stromal ablation, is presumed to play an important role in dry eye after LASIK (Wilson 2001; Ambrósio et al. 2008; Wilson and Ambrósio 2001).

We report a case of dry eye after LASIK in a highly disappointed patient, whose satisfaction improved tremendously after treatment of the ocular surface condition.

8.4.2 Case Report

A 43-year-old female was referred for a second opinion because of 'visual fluctuation and tired eyes associated with bad quality of vision' in both eyes. She had uncomplicated LASIK 4 months prior. Pre-operative medical records were unavailable, but she mentioned a moderate myopic astigmatic correction before suffering the surgical procedure. She was on artificial tears irregularly during the last months. UDVA was 20/40 OD and 20/30 OS. Manifest refraction was −0.75–0.75×145 OD, giving 20/30 and −1.00–0.75×85 OS, giving 20/25. Slit lamp bio-microscopy demonstrated a centred nasal LASIK flap hinge OU with a clear interface and no striae or corneal opacities. However, punctate epithelial erosions could be observed in both central and inferior corneal regions (Fig. 8.13) in both eyes as well as corneal staining of the corneal flaps. GAT was 11 mmHg OD and 8 mmHg OS at 11 a.m. and fundoscopic exam was unremarkable OU.

Figure 8.14 illustrates Placido disc-based anterior corneal topography axial maps, which reveals central corneal flattening OU suggesting a myopic treatment. Interestingly, the image of the Placido rings projected onto the cornea shows distortions and gaps in the mires, which is very suggestive of irregularity of the pre-corneal tear film. Ray-tracing aberrometry refraction maps evidenced a significant level of high-order aberrations in both eyes, especially coma and trefoil (Fig. 8.15), which is in accordance with the bad quality of vision referred by the patient.

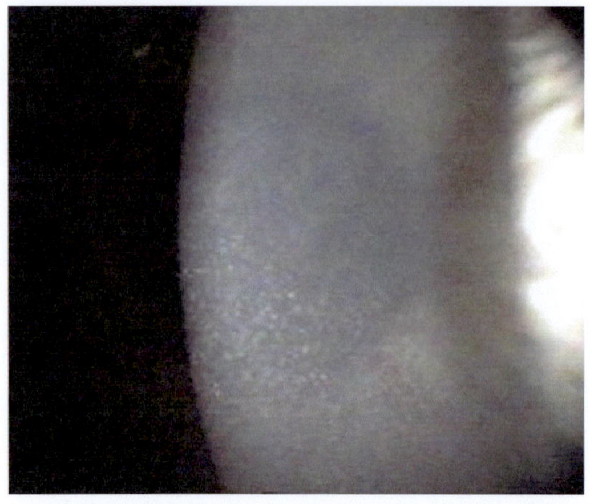

Fig. 8.13 Punctate epithelial erosions on the flap, including the area overlying the pupil

Based on these findings the diagnosis proposed was LASIK-associated dry eye, which could be evidenced by the presence of LINE typical findings. The treatment proposed was ocular surface optimisation with topical lubrication and omega-3 essential fatty acid (EFA) supplementation.

Three weeks after treatment, the patient mentioned a 'significant improvement in vision and eyes feeling better'. UDVA was 20/30 OD and 20/25 OS. By this time, manifest refraction was $-0.25-0.50\times152$ OD, giving 20/20 and plano -0.75×92 OS, giving 20/20. Slit lamp exam showed total absence of punctate epithelial erosions and improvement of tear film quality in

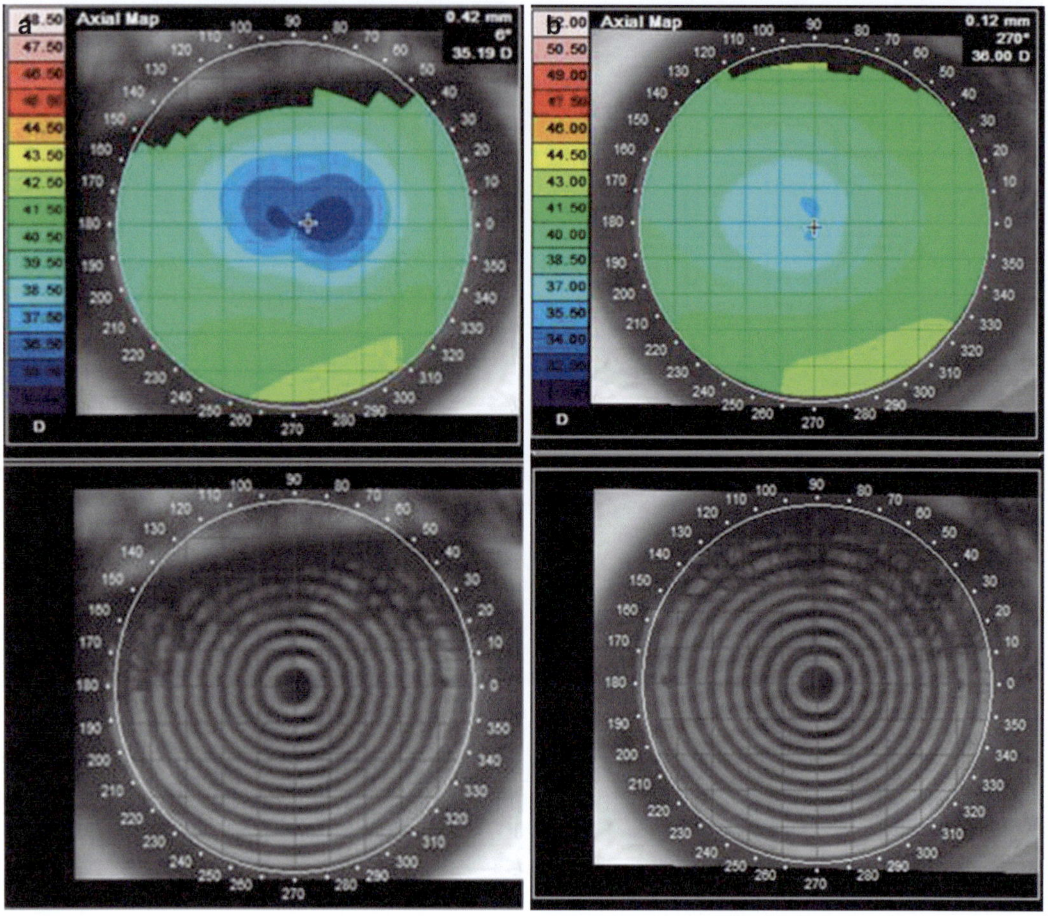

Fig. 8.14 Placido disc-based anterior corneal topography axial maps and reflex mires of Placido discs onto the cornea of OD (**a**) and OS (**b**). Note the gaps and distortions on the mires in OU

both eyes. This improvement was correlated with an improvement in quality of vision, what is objectively demonstrated by Fig. 8.16. This figure illustrates a comparison of both the auto-refraction and the simulated Snellen E maps, which simulates patient's vision according to the amount of aberrations, before and after treatment.

8.4.3   Discussion

LASIK-associated dry eye remains one of the major causes of patient dissatisfaction. This complication might interfere with quality of vision and is even thought to be associated with other complications such as regression (Wilson 2001). Many patients are not symptomatic, but subjective complaints about quality of vision can occur. Patient education and counselling along with an appropriate treatment to optimise the optical surface show improvement, but definitely, prevention is the best approach. Dysfunctional tear syndrome (DTS) is a complex and multi-factorial condition and is known to be a major risk factor for severe postoperative dry eye. It's critical to remember that a high percentage of patients self-select themselves for surgery because of difficulty in wearing contact lenses, and the major reason for this is underlying DTS.

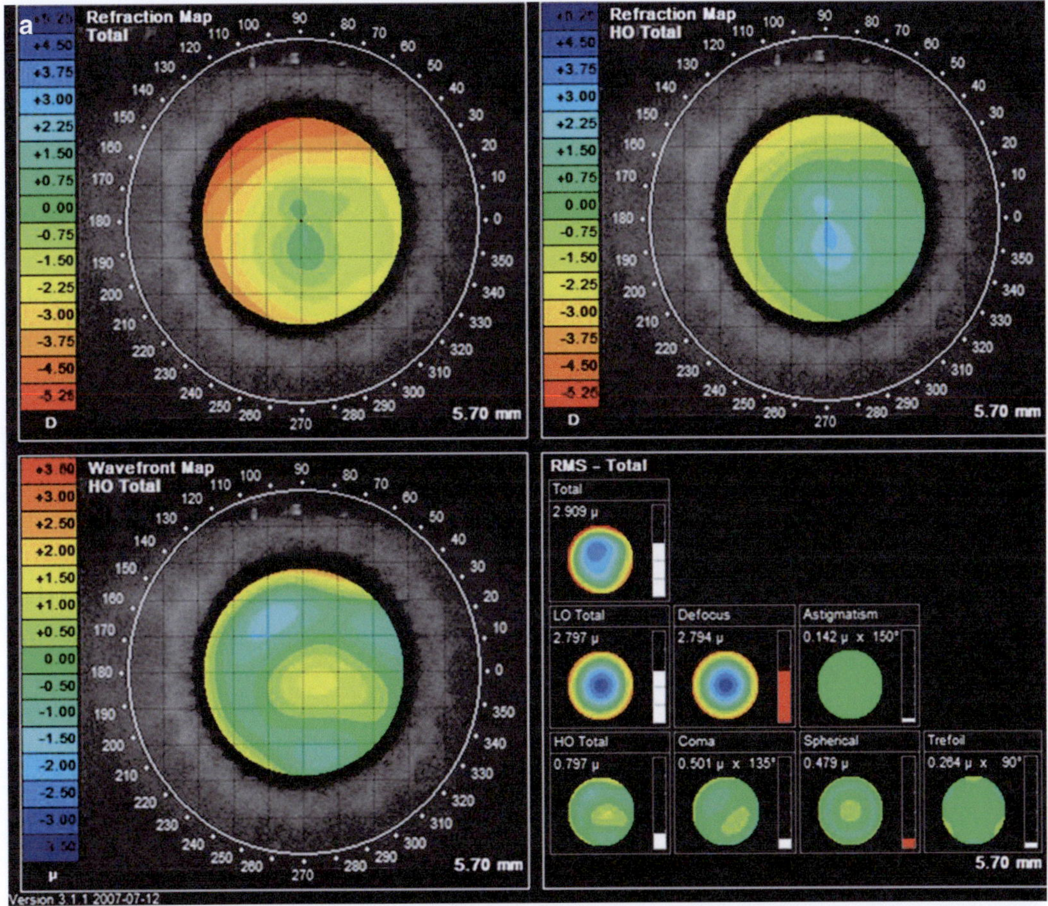

Fig. 8.15   Ray-tracing aberrometry refraction maps in OD (**a**) and OS (**b**) before treatment. A significant level of high-order aberrations in both eyes, especially coma and trefoil can be seen in OU

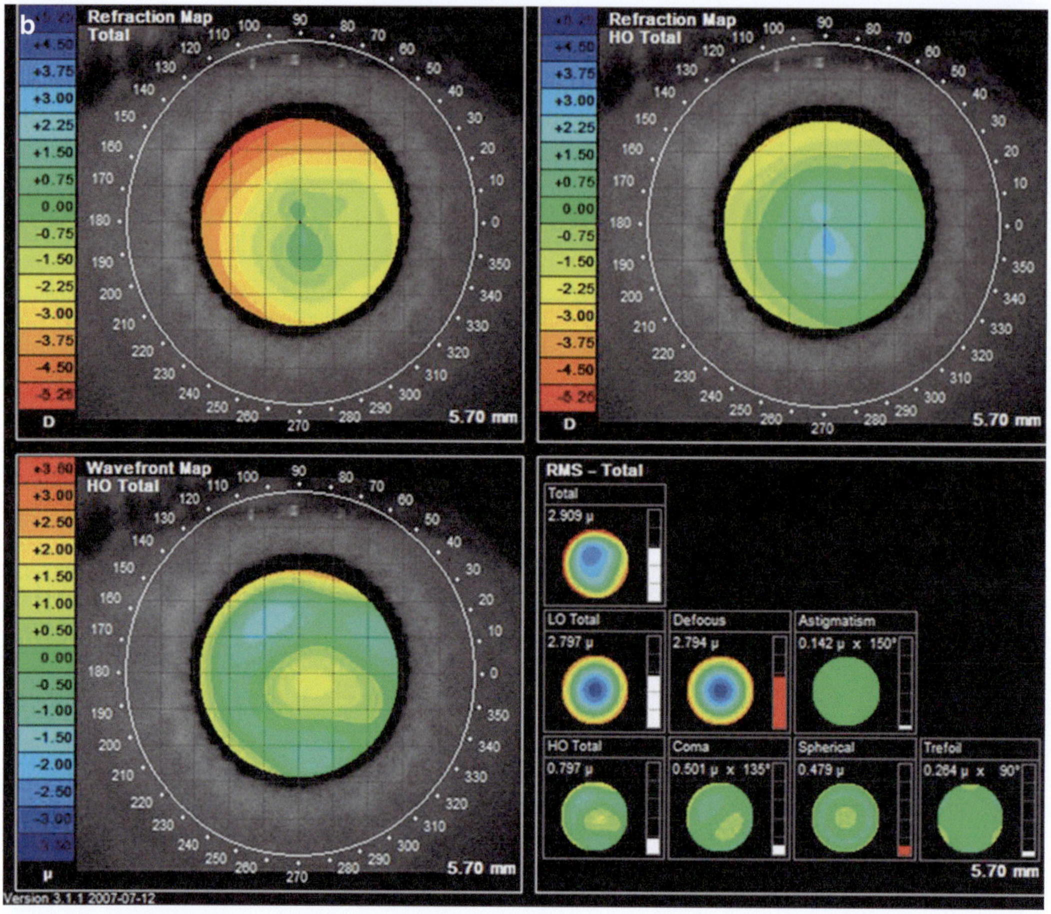

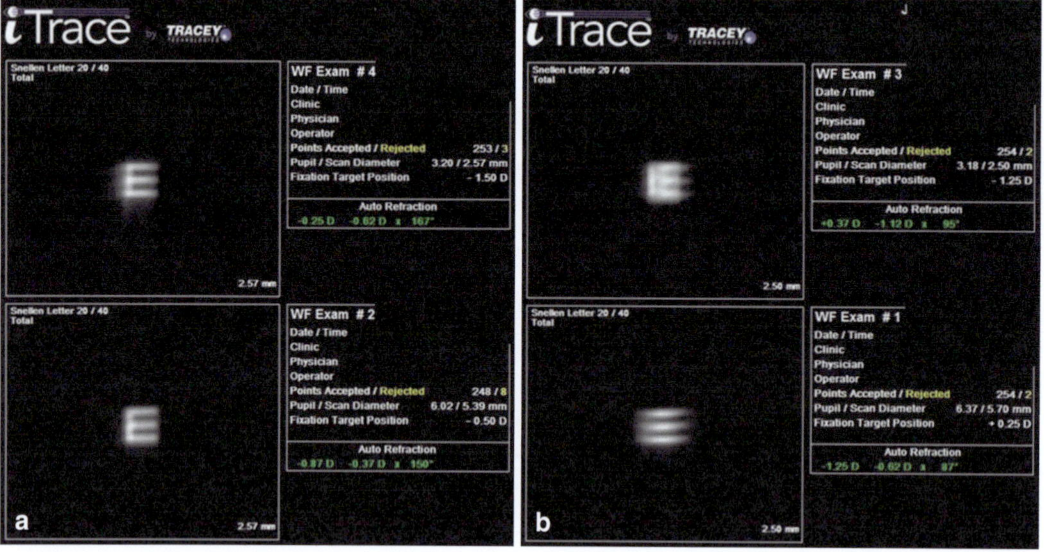

Fig. 8.15 (continued)

Fig. 8.16 Comparison of both the auto-refraction and the simulated Snellen E maps before (inferior) and after (superior) treatment in OD (**a**) and OS (**b**)

8.5 Medical Management of Dry Eye Case Report

Victor L. Caparas

8.5.1 Case Discussion

A 66-year-old man consulted with severe dry eye symptoms of grittiness, foreign body sensation, and severe ocular discomfort after reading for only a few minutes. He gave a two-and-a-half-year history of doctor shopping during which he went through, for varying lengths of time, a variety of dry eye medications, including steroids, cyclosporine and close to every commercial ocular lubricant available. On top of that, he had become dependent on vasoconstrictor drops to relieve his constant eye redness. He had been under treatment with a dermatologist for what he described was acne and which, after inspection, was clearly rosacea. He was also hypertensive, for which he was taking a diuretic and beta-blocker. Having given up on a cure for his dry eye, he had stopped all eye medications except for preserved carboxymethylcellulose drops which he applied almost every 20 min.

OSDI score was 93.8. Examination showed best-corrected vision of 20/25 for both eyes, conjunctival hyperaemia and severe corneal and conjunctival staining in both eyes. Tear film break-up time (BUT) was less than 2 s in each eye. Both eyes had a Schirmer I test of 4 mm. Lower lid tear meniscus was almost inexistent. His eyelid margins were thickened and vascularised, with areas of notching. Only 1–2 of the central meibomian orifices of both eyes were patent, all of which expressed cloudy secretions (Figs. 8.17, 8.18 and 8.19).

Points to Consider
1. Severe dry eye: severe symptoms and signs
2. Severe MGD
3. Rosacea

4. Medications with known dry eye implications
Ocular: vasoconstrictors, preserved lubricants
Systemic: diuretics, beta-blockers
5. No anti-inflammatory medication

Initial treatment regimen instituted was:
1. Fluorometholone drops, 3 times daily for 2 weeks only.
2. Cyclosporine 0.05 % drops, twice daily.
3. Doxycycline, 100 mg daily, as single dose.
4. Non-preserved lubricant drops.
5. Warm lid compresses, twice daily.
6. Omega-3 fatty acid diet supplement, 300 mg.
7. Modify systemic meds: substitute for beta-blocker/diuretic.
8. Discontinue vasoconstrictor drops.

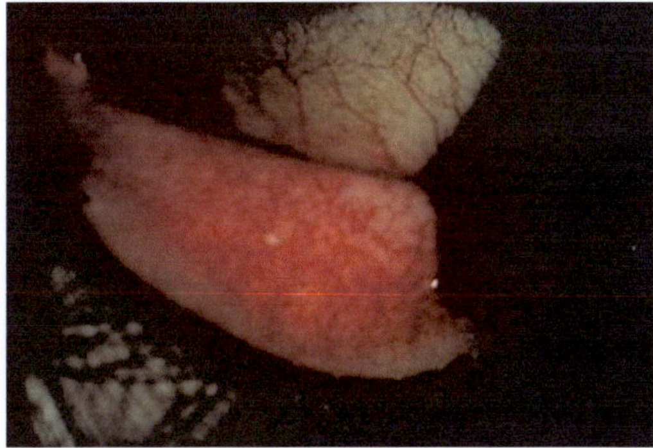

Fig. 8.17 Severely hyperaemic conjunctiva

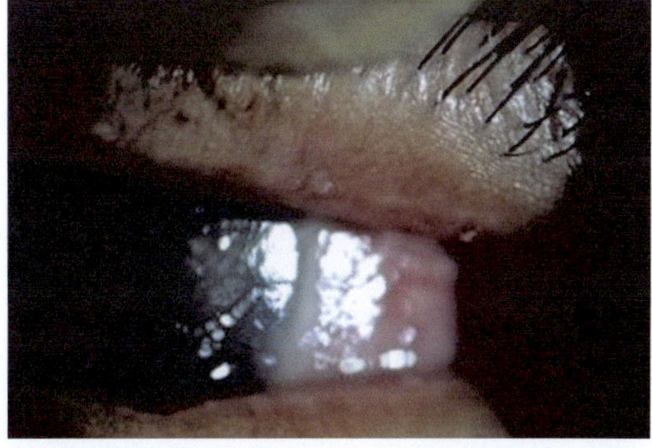

Fig. 8.18 Thickened and vascularised lid margin, opaque and scarred orifices

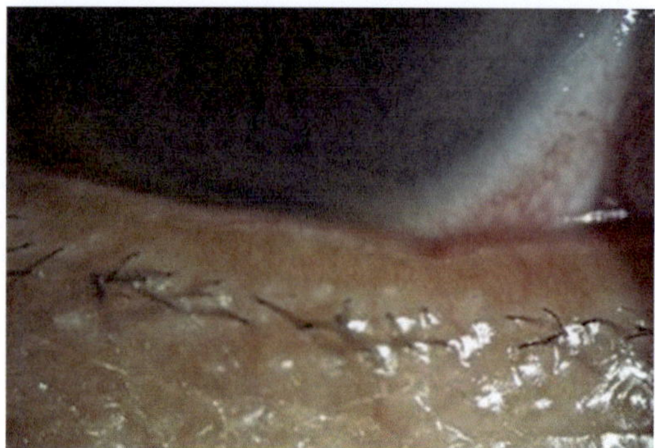

Fig. 8.19 Notching and ridging of lid margin

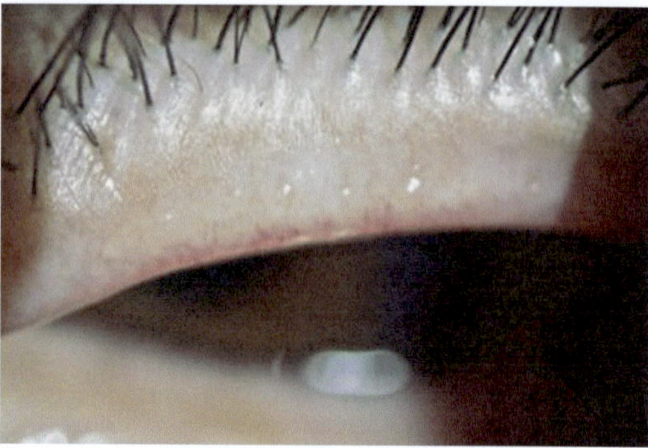

Fig. 8.20 Decreased vascularisation of lid margin, expression of slightly cloudy meibum from previously plugged orifices

9. Education: advised to avoid drafts, humidify air-conditioned environments, adjust reading/computer angle.
10. Advised patience!

Following 2 weeks of corticosteroid drops, the patient experienced slight symptomatic relief and mild alleviation of redness. After 3 months, OSDI score was 72.9, TBUT was up to 4 s, and a tear meniscus was visible. Ocular surface staining had decreased by 50 %. Still, the patient was uncomfortable and vocal about it, despite the improvement in objective signs. Following consultation, he was shifted to autologous serum, 8 times daily. Cyclosporine was discontinued temporarily and lubricants were allowed, as needed. Doxycycline, which was well tolerated, was continued on a month-to-month basis.

The patient tolerated well the autologous serum, and after 6 months of treatment, his condition improved slowly. (He, in fact, volunteered the information that the serum was a significant addition.) Staining of the cornea had disappeared, and that of the conjunctiva was minimal. TBUT increased to about 7 s and Schirmer to 7–8 mm. Lid margin inflammation was down, but the number of patent orifices and quality of expressed meibum had improved only marginally. His rosacea had also improved markedly. Despite improvement in objective tests, he continued to complain of foreign body sensation and having to blink very often. To supplement the volume of

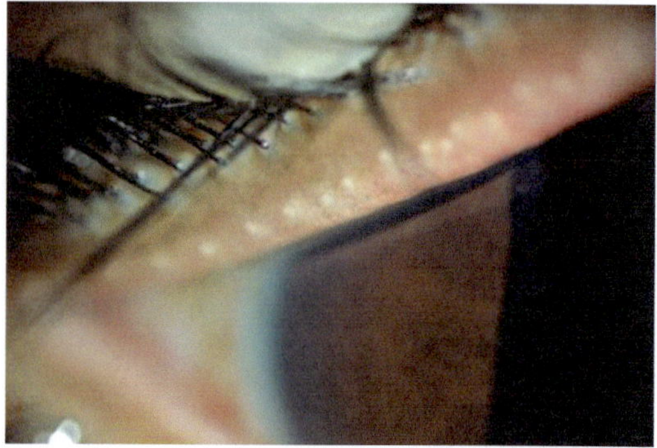

Fig. 8.21 Plugged orifices, granular to pasty meibum

tears, temporary collagen punctal plugs were inserted into both upper and lower puncta. Serum was continued, but to spare him from too many veni-punctures, this was alternated, roughly monthly, with cyclosporine. Although he had no adverse reactions, doxycycline was stopped temporarily.

After a full year under treatment, the patient claimed he was comfortable roughly half of the time. With some reservations, he could claim he was doing better than when he started. All measurable signs had improved significantly; however, the quantity and quality of his meibum was, at best, only slightly better. Lubricant use (non-preserved cellulose derivative alternated with an oil in emulsion) was down to about 6 times daily, with application of a gel at bedtime. Under normal conditions, both eyes were quiet and non-hyperaemic (Figs. 8.20 and 8.21).

Comment

1. Improvement in signs do not necessarily mean improvement in symptoms.
2. Dry eye condition improved with improvement in rosacea.
3. Serum appears to have contributed significantly to the improvement in the patient's condition and decreased dependence on lubricants.
4. The possibility of adverse effects of prolonged doxycycline use increases with duration of use, even if well tolerated initially, and therefore warrants discontinuation after several months of use.
5. Punctal plugs were inserted only when inflammation was controlled.
6. MGD improved less dramatically and continues to be a challenge in this patient.

8.6 Dry Eye: Future Directions and Research Case Report

Minako Kaido and Kazuo Tsubota

8.6.1 Case Report

A 44-year-old man with short BUT dry eye was administered the new ophthalmic solution of diquafosol tetrasodium. The subjective dry eye symptoms were alleviated 80 % after 1 month of the administration. The colour-coded map of higher-order aberrations (root mean square [RMS; mm]; 4.0 mm pupil) before (above) and at 1 month after (below) the administration of diquafosol tetrasodium ophthalmic solution is shown in Fig. 8.22. The reduction in higher-order aberrations and the stability of the colour-coded map were observed after the administration.

8.6.2 Case Report

A 59-year-old female with Sjögren's syndrome, using hyaluronate sodium solution and inserted

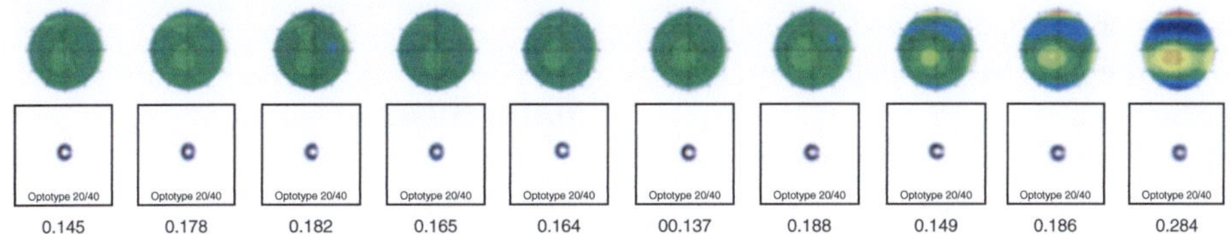

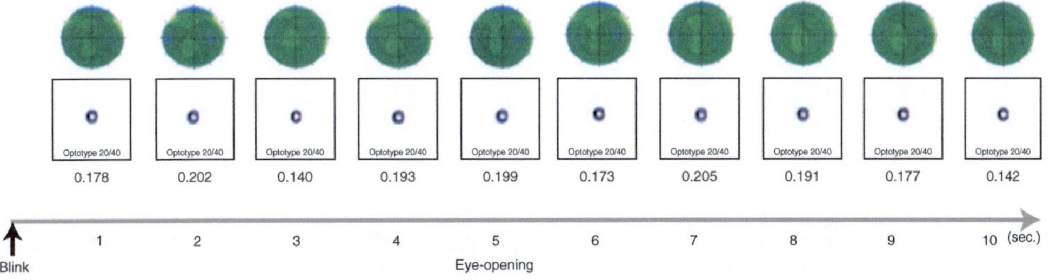

Fig. 8.22 A representative case of the diquafosol sodium ophthalmic solution administration. The reduction in higher-order aberrations and the stability of the colour-coded map were observed after the administration

Before the administration of rebamipide ophthalmic suspension

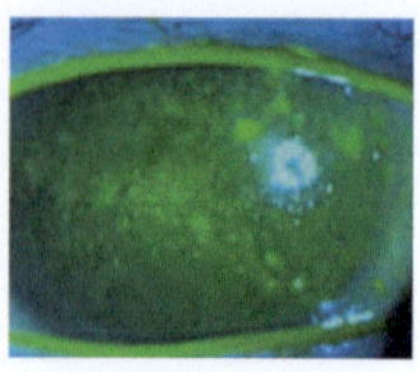
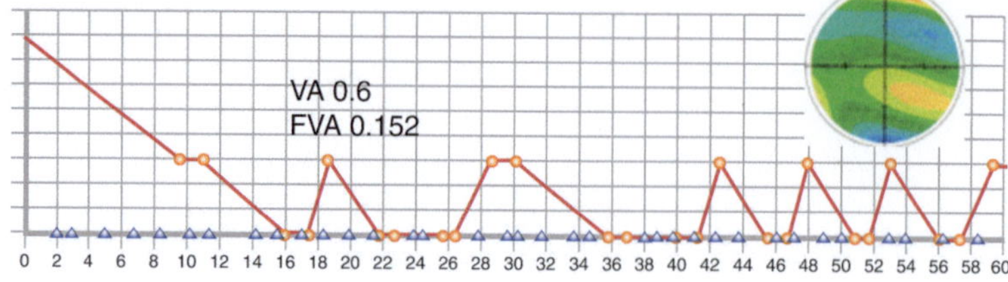

At 3 month after the administration of rebamipide ophthalmic suspension

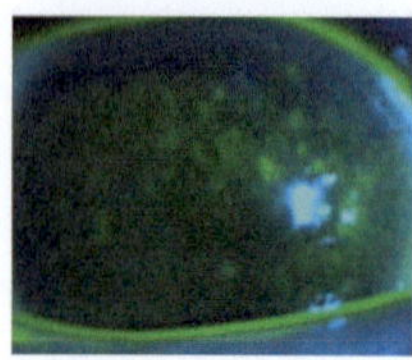
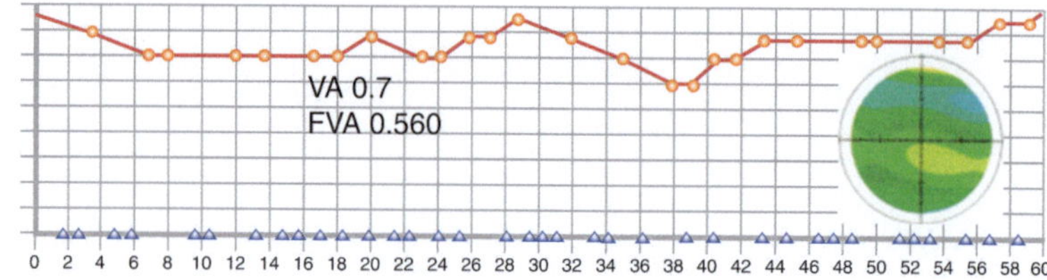

Fig. 8.23 A representative case of the administration of rebamipide ophthalmic suspension. Functional visual acuities were improved and higher-order aberrations were decreased at 3 months after the administration

lacrimal punctal plugs to upper and lower puncta, was additionally administered the new ophthalmic solution of rebamipide suspension. Superficial keratitis was improved after the administration.

Functional visual acuities were improved and higher-order aberrations were decreased at 3 months after the administration (Fig. 8.23).

Key Points

- Diquafosol tetrasodium and rebamipide are two novel potential treatments for dry eye disease.
- Dry eye disease can cause an increase in higher-order aberrations.
- Dry eye disease can cause a reduction in:
  - Best corrected visual acuity
  - Contrast sensitivity
  - Functional acuity (stability of vision in between blinks)

Compliance with Ethical Requirements Jennifer Craig, Colin Chan, Fernando Faria Correia, Issac Ramos, Marcella Salomao and Renato Ambrosio Jr. declare that they have no conflict of interest. Victor Caparas has received speaker's honoraria from Alcon and Allergan. He does not own any stock in either company. Kazuo Tsubota is a consultant for Santen Pharmaceutical Co., Ltd. Kazuo Tsubota has received research grants from Santen Pharmaceutical Co., Ltd.; Kowa Co., Ltd.; Otsuka Pharmaceutical Co., Ltd.; and JIN Co., Ltd. Kazuo Tsubota and Minako Kaido hold patent rights for the method and the apparatus used for the measurement of functional visual acuity (US patent no: 7470026).

All procedures followed were in accordance with the ethical standards of the responsible committee on human experimentation (institutional and national) and with the Helsinki Declaration of 1975, as revised in 2000 (5). Informed consent was obtained from all patients for being included in the study.

No animal studies were carried out by the authors for this article.

References

Alex A, Edwards A, Hays JD, Kerkstra M, Shih A, de Paiva CS, Pflugfelder SC (2013) Factors predicting the ocular surface response to desiccating environmental stress. Invest Ophthalmol Vis Sci 54:3325–3332

Ambrósio R Jr, Tervo T, Wilson SE (2008) LASIK-associated dry eye and neurotrophic epitheliopathy: pathophysiology and strategies for prevention and treatment. J Refract Surg 24:396–407

Bulbulia A, Shaik R, Khan N, Vayej S, Kistnasamy B, Page T (1995) Ocular health status of chemical industrial workers. Optom Vis Sci 72:233–240

Craig JP, Tomlinson A (1997) Importance of the lipid layer in human tear film stability and evaporation. Optom Vis Sci 74:8–13

Dougherty JM, McCulley JP, Silvany RE, Meyer DR (1991) The role of tetracycline in chronic blepharitis. Inhibition of lipase production in staphylococci. Invest Ophthalmol Vis Sci 32:2970–2975

Duffey RJ, Leaming D (2005) US trends in refractive surgery: 2004 ISRS/AAO Survey. J Refract Surg 21:742–748

Guillon JP, Guillon M (1993) Tear film examination of the contact lens patient. Optician 206:21–29

Hamrah P, Alipour F, Jiang S, Sohn JH, Foulks GN (2011) Optimizing evaluation of lissamine green parameters for ocular surface staining. Eye (Lond) 25:1429–1434

Henriquez AS, Korb DR (1981) Meibomian glands and contact lens wear. Br J Ophthalmol 65:108–111

Huo AP, Lin KC, Chou CT (2010) Predictive and prognostic value of antinuclear antibodies and rheumatoid factor in primary Sjogren's syndrome. Int J Rheum Dis 13:39–47

James MJ, Gibson RA, Cleland LG (2000) Dietary polyunsaturated fatty acids and inflammatory mediator production. Am J Clin Nutr 71:343S–348S

Knop E, Knop N, Millar T, Obata H, Sullivan DA (2011) The international workshop on meibomian gland dysfunction: report of the subcommittee on anatomy, physiology, and pathophysiology of the meibomian gland. Invest Ophthalmol Vis Sci 52:1938–1978

Korb DR, Blackie CA (2013a) Debridement-scaling: a new procedure that increases Meibomian gland function and reduces dry eye symptoms. Cornea 32:1554–1557

Korb DR, Blackie CA (2013b) Using goggles to increase periocular humidity and reduce dry eye symptoms. Eye Contact Lens 39:273–276

Mark KA, Sparacio RM, Voigt A, Marenus K, Sarnoff DS (2003) Objective and quantitative improvement of rosacea-associated erythema after intense pulsed light treatment. Dermatol Surg 29:600–604

Nichols KK, Nichols JJ, Mitchell GL (2004) The reliability and validity of McMonnies Dry Eye Index. Cornea 23:365–371

Olenik A, Jimenez-Alfaro I, Alejandre-Alba N, Mahillo-Fernandez I (2013) A randomized, double-masked study to evaluate the effect of omega-3 fatty acids supplementation in meibomian gland dysfunction. Clin Interv Aging 8:1133–1138

Schiffman RM, Christianson MD, Jacobsen G, Hirsch JD, Reis BL (2000) Reliability and validity of the Ocular Surface Disease Index. Arch Ophthalmol 118:615–621

Sobolewska B, Doycheva D, Deuter C, Pfeffer I, Schaller M, Zierhut M (2014) Treatment of ocular rosacea with once-daily low-dose doxycycline. Cornea 33:257–260

Toyos R, Buffa CM, Youngerman SM (2005) Dry eye and Sjogren's syndrome Case Reports. ASCRS EyeWorld

Wilson SE (2001) Laser in situ keratomileusis–induced (presumed) neurotrophic epitheliopathy. Ophthalmology 108:1082–1087

Wilson SE, Ambrósio R (2001) Laser in situ keratomileusis – induced neurotrophic epitheliopathy. Am J Ophthalmol 132:405–406